'Play Can Help' Series

LOOK AT IT THIS WAY

'Play Can Help' Series

LOOK AT IT THIS WAY

Toys and Activities for Children with a Visual Impairment

Roma Lear

Illustrated by Jill Hunter

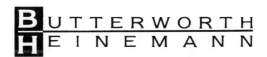
BUTTERWORTH
HEINEMANN

Butterworth-Heinemann
Linacre House, Jordan Hill, Oxford OX2 8DP
225 Wildwood Avenue, Woburn, MA 01801-2041

A division of Reed Educational and Professional Publishing Ltd

ℛ A member of the Reed Elsevier plc group

OXFORD   BOSTON   JOHANNESBURG
MELBOURNE   NEW DELHI   SINGAPORE

First published 1998

British Library Cataloguing in Publication Data
A catalogue record for this book is available from the British Library

ISBN 0 7506 3895 8

Typesetting by David Gregson Associates, Beccles, Suffolk
Printed and bound in Great Britain by Martins the Printers, Berwick upon Tweed

Contents

Acknowledgements

My grateful thanks to Jill Norris who started the first special needs toy library in the UK and founded the National Association of Toy and Leisure Libraries. She inspired us all to learn so much about the value of play and toys.

I am also indebted to:

All the children who, over the years, have unwittingly supplied the material for this book.

All the parents and therapists who have shared their ideas with me for the benefit of other children. You will find their names scattered throughout the book. The royalties earned from their contributions will benefit the National Association of Toy and Leisure Libraries.

All my toy library friends and the staff at NATLL for their encouragement, suggestions and advice.

Jill Hunter for her delightful illustrations, and Stuart Wynn-Jones, Anita Jackson and Caroline Gould for supplementary pictures.

Susan French for helping me to understand some of the problems faced by children with partial sight.

Ann Kirk for her good humoured and meticulous editing.

And particularly to Alison Wisbeach (Paediatric Occupational Therapist) for her invaluable advice and suggestions, and to my husband, John, who has acted as critic and sounding board throughout the writing of this book.

Disclaimer

Every effort has been made to ensure that the information contained in this book is as accurate, informed and up-to-date as possible at the time of going to press. The author and publisher cannot be held liable for any errors or omissions, nor for any consequences of using it.

Introduction to the 'Play Can Help' series

The toys and activities which appear in this series have been taken mainly from 'Play Helps', fourth edition. That book contains a collection of ideas relevant to children with widely differing play needs. In this series, those which will be particularly helpful to a child with a specific disability have been collected together in one volume. A few ideas may overlap into another book in the series. In addition, a number of new ones specific to the children in question have been added. No longer will the reader need to search all through 'Play Helps' to find a toy or activity to please an individual child. All that is needed is the right book in the 'Play Can Help' series!

This particular volume in the series deals specifically with play for children with a visual impairment, be they blind or with some degree of sight, however small. It also includes many play suggestions suitable for children with additional disabilities.

All the toys described need to be home-made by someone, but not necessarily by you!—within your family, circle of friends, local clubs for those who are retired, youth clubs, etc. I guess there are plenty of creative people with a little time to spare who would be delighted to help. There are several reasons for choosing to include only home-made toys and games. Designs in toy manufacture can change quickly and, by the time this book reaches you, a recommended toy may no longer be available. More importantly, I know from experience that a toy made with care for an individual child is sure to be a winner. With a little thought, it can be made just the right size and weight, and given an appropriate degree of difficulty; perhaps a few pieces for a beginner, more for a child who needs a challenge. It is no problem to make the toy extra strong, paint it in favourite colours or even add an enticing smell! Bought toys undoubtedly have an important part to play in the development of any child. Unfortunately, not every parent or carer has access to a good toy shop or toy library, and storage space can be at a premium. Some homemade toys (perhaps not intended to become family heirlooms, but just right for the age and stage of the child) can make a welcome and stimulating addition to a collection of playthings. There is also a place for some 'ephemeral' toys, not destined to last, but sure to be welcomed by a bored or sick child. (Useful on journeys and in hospital waiting rooms too!)

All the toys and games are in the low technology bracket and need only elementary skills for their construction. Some require only a pair of scissors and some PVA adhesive! Other materials used are either recycled, easily obtainable in the High Street, or by mail order (p. 4).

In the course of writing my earlier books, I met many professionals and others working in the field of Paediatrics. Frequently, they had original and valuable suggestions to offer. Relevant ones appear in this series under the name of the originator and the proportion of Royalties on these contributions will continue to be paid to the National Association of Toy and Leisure Libraries.

The 'Play Can Help' series is written mainly for parents and carers, but because of the number of ideas on offer, therapists and teachers may well find new ways of interesting and stimulating the children in their care. The book is all about having fun—with only a whiff of therapy!

In her Foreword to 'More Play Helps', Glenys Carter, the Director of NATLL neatly sums up my philosophy. She writes: 'The *process of play* is far more important than the toys. Parents and all practitioners working with children know that play is a child's work, through which they gain knowledge of themselves and of their world. The enjoyment, the excitement, the pride of achievement when new skills are mastered as the toys are used, and above all the quality of the interaction between adult and child are the real benefits.'

This volume, like all the others in the series, is divided into chapters, and for easy reference a full list of the contents is given at the beginning of each. Ideas for younger children come first.

The book is intended to be used rather as a collection of cookery recipes—not read from cover to cover. Dip into it now and then when you feel the need. I hope you will find plenty to tickle your palate!

January 1998   Roma Lear

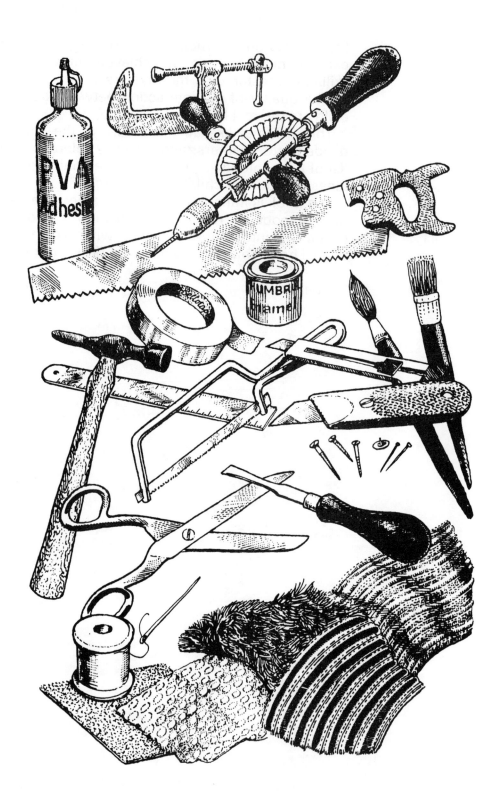

Before you begin

SOME HINTS ON TOYMAKING

The very first thing you must think about is *safety.* These days there are rigorous safety standards for manufactured toys, but even so I guess scarcely a week passes without the Casualty Department of your local hospital having to help a child in trouble through play. We all know how inquisitive children can be. Small fingers can soon stretch a little hole into a big one and innards that should be inaccessible are soon explored. They also have voracious appetites, and even if small pieces of toy are not eaten, they might easily be poked in ears or noses. Please consider the safety factor extra carefully if you make feely bags or rattles, and make sure you select contents that will be harmless if they are likely to escape.

Thankfully, most children emerge from childhood unscathed and this is due to the common sense and vigilance of their carers. They know the children's habits and steer them away from trouble! When making toys for children with special needs, an even larger dose of common sense is essential. A special cushion I once made for Sarah was stuffed with polystyrene chips—a material that should never be used with young children. But Sarah was long past the stage of putting things in her mouth, and her hands certainly did not have the strength to tear the cushion cover. Her cushion needed to be light and tactile. It was made specially for her as a 'one-off' toy, and I felt the rustling of the polystyrene chips might add to its attraction. The children around her were also passive and gentle, so there was no danger of her cushion falling into the wrong hands. The moral of this paragraph is—before you make any toy in this book consider what might happen to it! Perhaps you may need to modify the design, e.g. use lighter materials, if the toy is likely to be thrown, or make it heavier, if the child in question needs it to be made more stable.

When making a long-lasting toy always use the best materials available. The toy will look good, last longer and be a pleasure to make. Use birch plywood or Medium Density Fibreboard for wooden toys. Both sand down well, and you will avoid splinters or rough edges. New fabric is much stronger than some which has been through the wash many times. Use it double, or back it with calico for extra strength. Pay attention to seams. Stitch them twice and oversew to prevent them splitting. Sew buttons on *very* securely with strong button thread. PVA adhesive is excellent for sticking paper or card and is water-solvent if spilt. (A useful tip—if you spill some on a woollen garment, simply put it in the freezer overnight. In the morning you can pick off the brittle adhesive!) Poster paints, powder paints and felt pens sold as suitable for school use will be non-toxic. Humbrol enamel, sold in small pots for painting models, is safe for toys. It is made in lovely bright colours, covers most surfaces with only one coat and is quick drying. Polyurethane varnish is non-toxic when it is dry, and forms a good hard protective covering. Polyester fibre for stuffing soft toys is sold by the bag at craft shops and upholstery departments, etc. It should be labelled 'suitable for toy making' and marked with the CE safety mark.

The great advantage of making special toys—apart from the fun of it—is that they can be personalised for their user, and adapted to suit. Rattles and stability have already been touched upon, but perhaps a toy may need to be larger—or smaller; heavier—or lighter; made more simple—(make fewer pieces) or more difficult (increase the number). A toy can be thrown together as a five-minute wonder and soon end up in the bin, or it can be constructed with care and become a treasured possession which lasts for years. Circumstances alter cases, and the choice is yours.

All the toys in this book have been tried and tested with children, and all have proved their worth. Some have general appeal, others have been specially made to fill a particular play need, but all have been given the 'thumbs up' by the children. My less successful efforts have been discreetly carried away by the dustman!

SOME MATERIALS USED

Bells	From a craft or pet shop.
Buddies or Sticky Fixers	Small plastic pads with adhesive both sides.
Button thread	Strong, twisted, waxed thread. Used for mobiles, sewing on buttons.
Diffraction paper	A magical paper with a shiny surface. Hold it in different positions to catch the light, and wonderful patterns and colours are revealed. From Edu-Play (p. 4).
Dowel	Rod of wood, pine or ramin (stronger). Made in various thicknesses. From wood yards, DIY stores.
Dycem	A plastic sheet with special non-slip qualities. Can be ordered from Boots the Chemists or medical suppliers.
Fablon	Tough, sticky-backed plastic. Used for covering tables, etc. From DIY shops.
Fish grit	Used to cover the bottoms of aquaria. Sold by the bag at pet shops.
Magnetic tape	A strip of pliable, magnetised, rubber-like plastic, with an adhesive backing. Cut to size with scissors, peel off the protective

	paper and apply to toys as required. From educational suppliers and some DIY stores.
Magnets	Those used throughout this book are the disc kind. These are easier to stick to a toy than the horseshoe type, and keep their magnetism well if you remember to replace the 'keeper' on the face of the magnet after play. From craft shops.
Masking tape	A paper tape with a special adhesive, which does not damage paper and makes it easy to remove. From stationers.
Plastic foam	Used in upholstery. From specialist shops, street markets.

List of mail-order firms

All the materials used in making the toys are available in the High Street or DIY stores but, if personal shopping is difficult, here is a short list of mail-order firms which is up-to-date at time of publication.

Clear Vision Books
Clear Vision Project, Linden Lodge School, 61, Princes Way, London SW19 6JB
Tel: 0181 789 9575
    These books have a Braille version of the text inserted between the pages, so can be shared by children with a visual impairment and their sighted parents and friends.

Craft Depot
1, Canvin Court, Somerton Business Park, Somerton, Somerset TA11 6SB
Tel: 01458 274727
    For plastic canvas, touch'n play music buttons, squeakers, felt off-cuts, etc.

Edu-Play
Units H and I, Vulcan Business Centre, Vulcan Road, Leicester LE5 3EB
Tel: 0116 2625827
    For diffraction paper and bells.

Hope Education
Orb Hill, Huddersfield Road, Oldham, Lancashire OL4 2ST
Tel: 01616 336611
    For blank dice, scissors—various.

Just Fillings
Dept. PC, 1 Beechroyd, Pudsey, West Yorkshire LS28 8BH
Tel: 01274 691965
    For polyester fibre.

NES Arnold
Ludlow Hill Road, West Bridgford, Nottingham NG2 6HG
Tel: 01159 452201
    For general educational supplies and magnetic tape.

Nottingham Rehab
Ludlow Hill Road, West Bridgford, Nottingham NG2 6HD
Tel: 01159 452345
    For Dycem and special scissors for children.

Play for a child with a visual impairment

In the days when I was a Home Tutor, I needed to think about some of the problems which daily confront a child with little or no vision. The following lines are written for people who, like me at that time, may need to provide stimulating play without the benefit of professional advice. My newest pupil, Mary, was a girl of eleven who had recently and traumatically lost her sight. My brief from the Education Office was to try to help her (and her family) through these early days of readjustment, to remember that she would progress on to special education, and to make her schooling as normal as possible. This was my first experience of teaching a child with no sight at all and, at that time, there was no one to advise me on how to proceed. It seemed obvious that I should first try to understand how the child was feeling in her new and bewildering environment. I covered my head with a paper carrier bag and started to explore my home. The distance between the rooms was not at all as I expected, and I could not find the doors without running my fingers along the wall. Soon I realised my feet could detect the different floor coverings, and I could count the paces from here to there. After a few painful encounters with the furniture, I became cautious and used my arms like antennae. My paper bag experience lasted only a short while, but it was sufficient to give me a brief insight into Mary's new world. For a start, I knew she would appreciate things always being in the same place, and I realised I would have to take extra care in my use of words. To keep alive her memory of colour and size, I would need to include them in my descriptions, a detail I would not normally think about if I was teaching a sighted child.

Mary is now in full employment and, with the aid of her guide dog, leading a happy and interesting life. Since our days together, I have had the opportunity to play with many visually impaired children at the toy library. Some have never had useful vision. It can be difficult to remember that, unlike Mary, they have no idea of size, distance, speed, colour, etc.—all the information we normally pick up through our eyes. The young ones are often reluctant to stretch out when toys are pushed out of reach. Without adult encouragement and help, their playthings can stay that way. Older children tend to go for the toys they know, and may be reluctant to try something new unless it is introduced to them slowly and with plenty of explanation. Take, for example, a wooden construction set with its collection of bars, angles and wheels, which can be joined together with nuts and bolts. If this bewildering collection of pieces is simply tipped onto the table and the child is left to get on with it, I guess a frustrated and unhappy one will be the result. It is better to start with the pieces sorted into their compartments in the box. Then each one can be described and examined. Next, with the help of the child, a simple model is made. After this careful introduction, the chances are that his engineering skills will begin to emerge, and he will end up joining together several pieces all by himself—to his (and your) intense satisfaction!

To provide stimulating play for any child, it is essential to watch and listen, particularly for one who is still at the baby stage or has disabilities, which prevent him from selecting the toys of his choice. Perhaps he can tell you what he would like. If not, an inspired guess is necessary. Some children will play with one toy, such as a posting box, for a surprisingly long time. This can be a good thing if they really enjoy pushing the shapes through the correct holes—or it could be a bad thing, if it is because there is nothing more enticing on offer! Other children may discard a toy without fully realising its potential. I remember a blind boy (who also had severe learning difficulties) on one of the wards where I worked. At visiting time, his mother brought in a large beach ball. At first her son just pushed it away and showed little interest in it. Then she sat on the floor opposite him saying 'It's coming, Tony' and rolled the ball towards him. There were shrieks of delight when he successfully fielded it! He would never have bothered with the ball if his mother had not invented this simple game. To provide the right toy or activity at the right time is not an easy task, but it is a very rewarding one if, through play, the result is the development of a child's curiosity, confidence and knowledge.

Once child and toy are together, there is yet another way in which we can help. Make sure the child is in the best possible position to use his hands (and eyes) to best advantage. There must be many adults reading this book who remember with affection the BBC radio programme 'Listen With Mother'. To make sure the children were attending properly, every story time began with the question, 'Are you sitting comfortably? Then I'll begin'. The same principle applies to playtime. There are many ways of 'sitting comfortably'—perhaps with the child on your knee or on the floor between your legs; maybe in a playring or baby bath (p. 12), at a table or over a wedge. (Your therapist will advise as necessary.)

When making a toy or selecting one from a shop, it is wise to think about size. Small toys and those with many pieces are easily lost—a particular problem for the visually impaired. Colour may be important. Black and white give the greatest contrast, and can be more easily seen against, for instance, a heavily patterned carpet. Some children will go for bright primary colours while others prefer pastel shades. Another reason to watch and listen! An inbuilt sound makes a toy more attractive to some children; others are more interested in shapes and textures. Some children cannot bear the feel of certain fabrics, such as simulated fur though, in time, their opinion of it may change. Here again, watch carefully to find out what appeals at the moment and gradually try to extend the child's experience.

For the child with some sight, it is obvious that his play area must be well lit to make toys as visible as possible. Some children find it easier to distinguish the different parts of a toy if they are not jumbled up in a heap, but spread out a little, with gaps in between. A table with a matt surface or a cot sheet spread over the carpet may be helpful.

Perhaps this is the place to remind ourselves that a toy does not have to be expensive, or even to come from a toy shop at all. Every home is filled with exciting playthings—(but pick out the *safe* ones!) A visit to the kitchen will provide pans with lids to fit, baking trays to nest together, a wooden spoon to cut teeth on, a ring of measuring spoons to rattle about, unopened packets of dried goods to build with ... All splendid toys, and an excursion into Real Life!

Playtime can provide a perfect opportunity to help a visually impaired child develop his other senses. Suggestions for helpful toys and activities follow, but first let us consider the playneeds of very young or otherwise immobile children. Here a basic problem can be how to keep toys within reach. If you recognise this difficulty, read on for some simple solutions.

Making play possible

KEEPING TOYS WITHIN REACH

Suspending toys for children who are lying down

The following devices should be positioned within easy reach of the child's hands so that he can biff, grab, grasp and let go as he pleases. The suspended toys are intended to be played with when baby is on his own and probably unsupervised so *remember the safety factor* and select as appropriate.

An Elastic Luggage Strap

Instant

This has strong hooks on both ends and can be hung across the cot so that the child can biff and grab the toys that dangle from it. It can easily be removed when the cot side needs lowering. It should be *slightly* stretched between the cot rails, so it is wise to measure before buying. Hang some toys with tape or string, but use elastic for others so that when they are pulled and released, they will bob about.

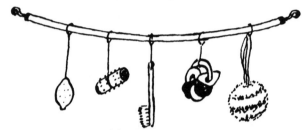

An Elastic Washing Line

Instant

Jeanette Maybanks

Here is an easy but effective way of suspending toys at any height. The brainwave came from a busy Mum who wanted to amuse her baby while he was still at the precrawling stage and floorbound on a rug. The idea could be used to hang toys within reach of any child who needs to play in a similar position. Just hang a length of elastic between two suitable points—the rungs of chairs might do. At intervals along it, attach strong bulldog clips. (These are obtainable from large stationers and office equipment suppliers.) As the name suggests, these clips grip very firmly and will withstand a fair amount of tugging. From the clips, dangle any old thing, perhaps a handkerchief, or a fluorescent sock with a rattle in the toe, a soft toy on a piece of ribbon or a glove with a little bell in a finger.

A Plastic Garden Chain

*Instant
(and long-lasting)*

Here is another way of stringing toys in a row, either for a child in a cot, or for one lying on the floor. The chain looks attractive and, of course, is very strong—and washable! When it is firmly fixed in position, simply tie the toys to the links, position the child comfortably and let her have a go.

Goal Posts

Long-lasting

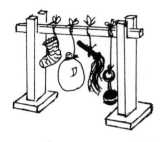

A Hotch-Potch of Toys to Biff, Grab or Pull

Instant

Suggested by
Christine Cousins,
Judy Denziloe,
Margaret Gilmore,
Lilli Nielson and
Fiona Priest

This idea is borrowed from the football pitch. A child can lie between the posts and reach all the delights that dangle from the crossbar. The posts are slotted (or fixed with brackets) to sturdy feet so that the whole frame is very stable. The crossbar rests in grooves cut in the top of the posts and, at the end of playtime, the whole contraption can be taken apart for easy storage.

Here are some suggestions:

- Balloons. Sausage-shaped ones are easier to hit. A few grains of rice inside, or a small bell or two, make them even more exciting. Do not fully inflate—to reduce the risk of popping.
- A bunch of ribbons or strips of non-fray material firmly tied together.
- Any plastic bottle with a handle, that once contained a non-toxic liquid. Put inside something safe that will rattle. Before hanging up, fix on the lid with a dab of plastic glue, like U-Hu.
- A sock with something securely tied in the toe—a rattle, fir cone, squeaky toy ...
- A string of *large* buttons, perhaps with a bell (from the pet shop) added here and there.
- Hang what you already have—a soft toy perhaps. Suspend it from a length of strong elastic, so that it will bob about if pulled and released.
- See if a plastic baby mirror appeals. This is large and shiny and has convenient holes in the frame from which to hang it.
- Hang up a *bunch* of rattles—much easier for a child to see, and biff and grab than a single one hung up on its own.
- Thread-coloured cotton reels or till reels on a string or loop. Make sure they cannot be pulled off.
- Use the lid of a treacle tin with a small hole punched near the rim. This lid is strong, shiny and has a well-turned edge. To make its rotations more dramatic, stick a circle of brightly-coloured Fablon on one side, or hang two or three closely together, so that if one is touched it will knock against the others.
- Hang up an empty wine bag from a box of wine. Inflate it and, perhaps, decorate it with some plastic stickers.

See also
Dancing Danglement, p. 52
A Bamboo Mobile, p. 52
A Ship's Bell Rattle, p. 59
Octopully, p. 63
A Friendly Rattlesnake, p. 66. Attach strings.
Grab Bags, p. 86
Amorphous Beanbag, p. 88. Attach strings.
A Manx Feely Cushion, p. 89. Attach strings.

For children who are just starting to sit up

Play Necklace for an Adult to Wear

Instant

When playing with very young (and possibly floppy) children at the toy library, I find it difficult to hold them securely and, at the same time, offer them interesting toys of the rattle variety. I manage beautifully if I bedizon myself with a 'play necklace'. This is just a loop of soft material, for my comfort, not string which would cut into my neck if the baby tugged. I attach rattles, squeaky toys, etc. at intervals around the loop and away we go!

Playing in a Baby Bath

Instant

Pam Courtney,
Teacher of Visually
Impaired Children

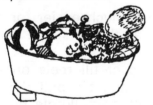

For a *small* child who is able to sit up, a baby bath with one end slightly raised makes a good 'child and toy container'. The high sides of the bath also help to keep toys to hand. Pam has found that, for some children, it is better to put plenty of toys in the bath—not just one or two. This bonanza cannot be ignored and should tempt the child to investigate—and play. As an alternative to a baby bath, you might use a plastic laundry basket. This has the added advantage that toys can be strung across it or tied to the sides—useful if the child might otherwise end up sitting on them.

A Play Bag

Instant

Use an old handbag with an easy opening. Put a toy or two inside, and some safe junk like a small sock with a cat ball (from the pet shop) in the toe.

Long-lasting

Make a special bag to hold toys. One which incorporates buttons, zips, etc. is described under 'Dressing

Skills', p. 111 but that version is too complicated for a child who is just beginning to sit up. All you need at this stage is a bag with a circular base, like an old-fashioned Dorothy Bag. If the base is stiffened with a circle of cardboard (made removable if the bag is likely to go in the washing machine), it will sit nicely on the floor. To give the bag guaranteed child appeal, add patch pockets here and there, both *inside* and *out*. These will be easier for the child to find if made from materials of different textures. Add a hem and a draw-string to the top of the bag and, at the end of playtime, all the toys can be stored away tidily until next time.

A Junk Box

Instant

Every child should have one! A magical collection of bits and bobs kept in a special container, (such as a plastic ice cream tub or strong cardboard carton) costs nothing, and can be the best toy ever. We have all known children who have ignored an expensive toy, but spent ages playing with the box or the wrapping paper. A Junk Box capitalises on this kind of play. It is nothing more than a collection of *safe* rubbish—perhaps a large piece of bubbly plastic, a short length of thick (unswallowable) metal chain, some empty cotton reels, some packaging from a box of jam tarts, a real carrot or a lemon ... the list can go on and on, always subject to the *safety factor* and the age and habits of the child—and possibly his playmates. The contents of the box can be changed as often as fresh delights occur to you. It can bridge the gap between boredom and being overwhelmed by new experiences. Its appeal may last well into later childhood as its contents are updated and it becomes a 3D box of memories—perhaps containing shells brought home from a holiday, or presents which are a reminder of a special occasion. If you think about its contents, you can have an enormous influence on your child's incidental learning through play. Always describe and explore together new items when you introduce them to the box. It is so easy to think that an object so familiar to you is also well known to the child. When the Junk Box becomes too full, watch carefully to see which items he always goes for and, if possible, have his permission, before you remove anything. That tatty bit of well-sucked blanket may be his most treasured possession, and a real source of comfort when he is feeling lonely.

For children playing at a table

A Tabletop Necklace

Quick

Mrs Crane, Teacher,
The Manor School

Tying toys to a necklace for a *child* to wear is obviously not a good idea, because of the risk of it tightening round his neck. But to make a string of playthings which can be looped over a tabletop is a safe way of keeping toys within reach.

The first tabletop necklace I came across was made —in desperation—by a teacher in a school for children with severe learning difficulties. In her group were several lively lads, and one who was not able to move from his wheelchair. This boy was quiet and gentle. His favourite occupation was to shake and rattle plastic toys. Unfortunately, his class mates often took a fancy to his playthings and grabbed them from him, leaving him very upset. (Naturally!) His teacher came up with this answer. She collected all his favourite toys and tied each to the middle of a strip of nylon tape (scrap from a factory). She cut three more pieces of the same tape, each three times the width of the play table. She plaited these together and, at intervals, both ends of the tape with a toy attached were incorporated into the plait.

This long 'necklace' was laid across the tabletop and passed under it so that the ends could be knotted together to make a loop. The boy could now sit at the table and pull the necklace towards him until he reached the toy of his choice. He might go for 'Flip Fingers', a large plastic ring with strings of buttons attached, a plastic car, a pair of plastic scissors, a trainer ball with holes in it and a bell inside, a string of large beads, a bunch of keys or various rattles. At last he could enjoy his favourite activity in uninterrupted peace.

Note
If this idea appeals to you, a simple way of making a similar tabletop necklace is to use a length of plastic

garden chain. Buy sufficient to wrap loosely round the top of the play table. Lie the chain over the top and join the ends together with string. Now all the 'necklace' needs is some toys tied to it at suitable intervals – not too close or they will tangle together. Remember to change the toys now and then!

A Play Box

Quick

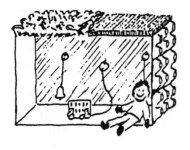

This useful device serves two purposes. It keeps toys within reach and the textured outside encourages small fingers to explore the shape, giving the child an idea of the size of the play area.

Stick some interesting textures to the outside of the box. For ideas, turn to page 91. Make holes in the sides here and there and fix loops of elastic to them. Double the elastic in half, tie a knot to form the loop, then poke the two ends through the hole. Tie a *large* knot—that will not pull through—on the outside of the box. Tie toys to the loops. The floor of the box makes a useful surface for building games because the bricks cannot topple out of reach.

For children playing in the car

A Play Pinny

Quick

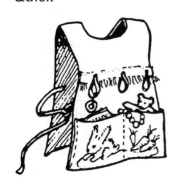

Over the years our toy library at Kingston-upon-Thames has been supplying pinnies of an appropriate size to children with visual or physical problems. With the help of this useful little cover-up, toys attached to the loops cannot be dropped or pushed out of reach. On a long journey, a play pinny can be a boon to any small child strapped in his safety seat, possibly with no-one beside him to retrieve dropped playthings. The pinny ensures that child and toys stay together!

The basic pattern is just an oblong of material, the width of the child's shoulders, with a hole cut in the middle for his head to go through. A pocket is made along the bottom of the front. It is divided down the middle with a row of stitching to make a separate pocket for each hand. Three loops of tape are sewn to the front of the pinny. It is wise to stitch a reinforcing strip behind these, and attach them very securely. They will have to withstand a considerable amount of pulling and tweaking. The raw edges are neatened by binding round the neck and hemming the top of the pocket, sides and bottom of the back. Short lengths of tape are stitched to each side. When these are tied together, they stop the pinny from rucking up when worn. Now all that is needed are some little surprises to hide in the pockets, (crunchy paper, a fir cone?) and some suitable toys to tie to the loops of tape (rattle, teether, soft toy?).

For children who tend to scatter their toys

A Picture Frame

Instant

Jenny Buckle,
Play Leader and Parent

It is so easy for Lego bricks, Play People with all their accessories—or any other toy with lots of small pieces—to be scattered over the tabletop, but put them inside a picture frame and the problem is solved!

This idea is particularly useful for older children with limited reach.

A Meat Tin

Instant

This 'toy container' has the obvious advantage of a high lip and can make a useful play area for children lying over a wedge. A piece of black felt glued to the bottom will help the toys to show up. It will also prevent any distracting shine from the tin and stop toys from sliding around.

Magnetic Tape and a Metal Playboard

Quick

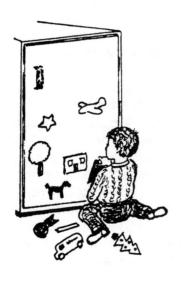

This method is fun for all children, but it is particularly *useful* for those with a visual handicap or poor hand-eye coordination. Play pieces with the magnetic tape applied will stick to the board until the child chooses to move them. It is even possible to make the adhesion light or firm, according to the amount of magnetic tape that is applied.

Magnetic tape can always be obtained from Educational Suppliers (p. 4) and can sometimes be found in High Street shops. It is sold by length and comes in ribbon form with a self-adhesive backing. Cut off the required length and stick it to the underside of small toys, mosaic shapes for pattern making, 'push together puzzles', or what you will.

Provide a metal playboard from a toy shop, usually sold complete with letters, numbers and shapes. A large, shallow biscuit-baking tray works just as well, but this is lighter and will probably need anchoring down. The best metal playboard on offer may well be the front of the fridge!

Learning to look

THIS CHAPTER IS FOR CHILDREN with some degree of sight, however small. A Therapist who works with visually impaired children tells me that they often need to be taught the three basic ways of using their vision:
1. To focus on a fixed object (keeping their eyes still).
2. To follow (track) a moving object (controlling their eye movement).
3. To scan a group of objects in order to identify a specific one (making full use of whatever vision they have).

This careful approach to 'looking' may be particularly important for a child with additional disabilities. The ideas which follow are grouped under one of these three categories.

LEARNING TO FOCUS ON A FIXED OBJECT

Here are some 'instant' ideas for ringing the changes. They are intended to be held by an adult at an appropriate distance for the child to see. They are *not* toys for children to handle.

1. *Tinsel ball.* Wind up some Christmas tinsel into a ball and tuck in the end. (Bind the ball with cotton if you think it may come unrolled.) Attach a string. Hold it *still*, but set it spinning so that it catches the light.
2. *Wine bag.* Tie a string to the stopper of the silver bag from the inside of an empty wine box. Slightly inflate it. Perhaps decorate it with strips of black adhesive tape.
3. *Drinks can.* Hang an empty drinks can from a string. Tie a large button, or some matches, or a small twig, etc. to one end of the string. Post this end through the hole in the can. As you hold the can by the string, the bottom end will wedge inside the lid and the can will hang at an angle. Decorate it, or not, to suit your fancy. If a child's attention is not immediately captured, try tapping the tin gently.
4. *Birthday candles.* Candles on a birthday cake always rivet the attention of the guests. With a keen eye to safety, try a larger candle flame. Candles in holders set in tins are easily available in the High Street. Of course blowing out the candle is part of the fun!
5. *Torch beam.* In a darkened room, shine a torch beam on the wall.

When you first make the acquaintance of a new baby, what do you do? I guess you call his name, smile, nod your head, and generally make your face as noticeable as you can! It was Dr Elizabeth Newson, speaking at a toy library meeting several years ago, who made us realise that Mum (or Dad!) is the baby's first and best toy. The face of a caring adult has all the essentials—colour, movement, sound and *surprise*. The teeth appear, then hide; the tongue too; the eyes open and shut, and the mouth changes shape and makes odd noises like 'Boo!' Anything can happen! Pop-up toys also have all these essentials, plus a certain therapeutic value. Held by an adult, they can help a baby direct his gaze this way and that, up or down, left or right. When the child is able to hold the toy for himself, he will need to use both hands to make it work. While playing he should learn all about 'in' and 'out' and how to surprise people!

TOYS TO ENCOURAGE LOOKING AT A FIXED OBJECT

A CD Mobile

Quick and long-lasting

Carole Sunter,
Teacher of Visually
Impaired Children,
Orkney

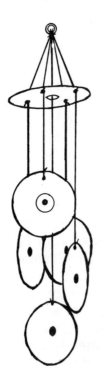

Here, at last, is a special mobile for children with low vision. As it is made from unwanted compact discs, it catches the light beautifully and reflects its rainbow patterns on nearby walls. The large surface area of each hanging CD helps it to rotate and sway in the slightest air current. Should two bump together, the gentle noise they make is an added attraction.

Materials
- Old CDs, say six, as in the picture.
- Small drill bit.
- Fishing line, or strong thread.
- Curtain ring for the hanging loop.

Method
Choose one CD to be the spacer disc at the top of the mobile. If it only has one shiny surface, make sure this is on the under side when the mobile is assembled. Drill four small, equidistant holes near the circumference of the spacer disc. (Use a *small* drill bit or, Carole says, the disc may shatter.) Drill one small hole near the circumference of each of the other five discs. Attach a fairly long hanging string to each one. Cut off any surplus once your finished mobile is hanging as you want it. Assemble the mobile as illustrated.

The easiest way to do this is to tie a string to the curtain ring, If no-one is handy to hold it for you, rest a stick (broom handle?) between the backs of two upright chairs and suspend the curtain ring from that. Thread a hanging string with a disc attached through the centre of the spacer disc. Tie it firmly to the curtain ring. (At this stage the spacer disc will flop over it.) Poke the thread of another disc through one of the outer holes of the spacer disc. Wind the thread over the edge of the disc and up through the hole again. Adjust the height so that the disc hanging through the centre of the spacer disc is now dangling clear and tie the side string to the curtain ring. Repeat the process for the other three discs. Hang them at different levels for the best effect and freedom of movement. Ease the spacer disc nearer to the curtain ring. The weight of the four discs suspended round the edge will now keep it in position. Hang this attractive, glittery mobile in a slight draft, and where it will catch the light.

Pop-up Dolly

Quick

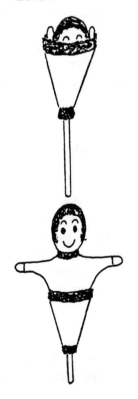

This toy is colourful and strong, and will withstand all but the most determined teethers.

Materials
- A wooden spoon. It *must* have a long handle if the dolly is to pop up properly.
- A cardboard or plastic cone from a spool of wool used on a knitting machine.
- Humbrol enamel in suitable colours for the face.
- A small piece of *thin* material for the dress.
- Thicker material to cover the cone.
- Scraps of trimming for decoration.
- PVA adhesive, needle and thread.

Method
Start by painting the face on the bowl of the spoon. Place the eyes in the middle and a smiley mouth below. Paint the back and inside edge of the bowl to represent hair. While the paint is drying, cut out the dress from the thin material. Fold it in half and cut out a shape like a flat letter T. Make sure that when the sides are sewn up, the bottom will be wide enough to fit comfortably round the top of the cone. Stitch up the side seams and turn the dress right side out. Cut out two small felt hands (as in the illustra-

tion), turn in the raw edges at the ends of the sleeves and sew in the hands. Now make a neck opening just large enough for the handle of the spoon to go through. Stick the dress to the spoon, just below the bowl. Use PVA adhesive generously and bind round the neck with cotton for extra strength and to prevent the dress from pulling away from the neck before the adhesive has set. Thread the handle of the spoon down through the hole in the cone. Hold the dress round the outside of the lip of the cone. Check that the dolly completely disappears inside, and will pop up and down properly. You may have to shorten the skirt if it is too bulky, but beware of cutting away too much—a mini skirt will not allow the dolly to hide inside the cone. Stick the skirt securely to the lip of the cone and bind it with cotton as for the neck. Cover the cone with thick material. (Stick and/or sew.) Felt is ideal as it will not fray. For extra strength, it is worthwhile sewing the hem of the dress to the cover and neatening the join with velvet ribbon, or lampshade trimming, etc. Embellish the neck with a ruff of gathered lace or ribbon.

Pop-up Matchbox

Quick

Marianne Willemsen-van Witsen

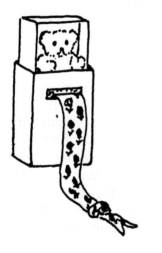

The illustration explains this toy. Just pull the ribbon, and the tray of the matchbox will rise most of the way out of its cover to reveal its hidden treasure.

Materials
- A matchbox.
- A short length of ribbon, about 2cm wide.
- A bead (optional).
- A decorative cover for the matchbox.
- Something to stick inside for the surprise—a tiny doll, a toy from a cracker, or perhaps a familiar face cut from a photograph. If you have time and the inclination, you might create a little scene inside the tray, such as a window looking out onto a country scene, with dainty lace curtains and pot plants on the window sill!

Method
Remove the tray from the matchbox cover. Cut a slot about 2cm from the top of the cover (wide enough to

take the ribbon). If you make it nearer the top, the tray will come right out when the ribbon is pulled. If you make it further down, not enough of the tray will rise up. Even making a simple little toy like this can have its technical hazards!

Thread the ribbon through the slot to the inside of the cover, and pull it up and over the back. Stick it along the entire length of the back. Insert the tray gently so that it sits in the ribbon sling, then press it down. (The ribbon will shorten as the tray disappears inside the cover.) Tie a bead to the free end of the ribbon. Pull it gently to make sure the toy is working properly and the tray rises up as you expect.

Take the tray out and decorate the part that will show. Then decorate the cover—the quickest way is to wrap it in coloured Sellotape, and this will also cover the abrasive strips at the side.

Jumping Jacks

Long-lasting

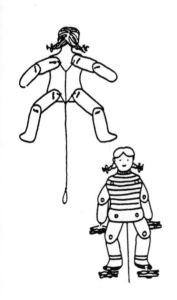

Jumping Jacks are traditional toys, usually made in wood. This version is in cardboard. It combines movement with sound, and is jointed with paper fasteners—the kind with 'legs' that open out.

It is sensible to make a paper pattern first. This can help you to decide on the size and the shape of the pieces, and you can make sure your design will work well before you spend time on the cardboard version.

Before you begin, look at the illustration and work out the mechanics of making your Jack (or Jill) jump. Then draw the body with the head attached by a fairly thick neck (for strength). Cut out two sausage-shaped arms and decide on the best positions for them. They must swivel on the paper fasteners so as to be horizontal with the body when the connecting string is pulled fully down, and be almost hidden by the body when relaxed. Cut out the legs, also sausage-shaped, but larger than the arms and with suggested feet on the end. When you are happy with your design, transfer the shapes to fairly thick cardboard and cut them out with a craft knife or Snips (really strong kitchen scissors similar to secateurs). Paint all the pieces. Fix on the limbs with paper fasteners, and string them as shown in the illustration. For an added attraction, tie a string of foil milk-

23

bottle tops (with a button on the bottom of the string to stop them slipping off), to the hands and feet. Alternatively, tie on bells.

Hang your Jumping Jack against a plain wall if possible, and just out of a child's reach, so that the string must be pulled to make him dance.

Plywood Owl Jumping Jack

Long-lasting

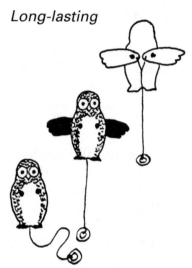

This toy works on the same principle as the one above, but only his wings move. If you have a fretsaw, it is easy to make, and the finished owl is very robust.

Make a paper pattern first. Draw the owl's head and body, making him about 30cm (12") long. Give him large eyes and make him chubby so that his wings will fold neatly behind his body when at rest. Draw his wings and try them out by fixing them in place with paper clips. Make sure they will flap nicely. Transfer the body and wing shapes to the plywood and cut them out. Sandpaper all the parts and paint in the eyes, beak and feathers. Drill two holes in each wing, one to fix it to the body and the other near the edge for the pull string. I joined my wings to the body with piping cord, knotting it in front of the body and behind the wings. Small nuts and bolts or rivets could be used. String up as shown in the illustration.

Note
After several weeks of heavy use, the piping cord on my owl stretched, and the wings started to rotate(!) causing a tangle at the back. Should this happen to you, the remedy is easy. Just glue a small strip of wood across the owl's shoulders to act as a stop.

Visi-bottles

What happens to your empty bubblebath bottle before it lands up in the dustbin? In our house, I used to half fill it with water and give it to our energetic little two-year-old. He would use it like a cocktail shaker to build up an impressive head of bubbles inside the bottle, then watch intently as they gradually popped, restoring the water to its previous state and ready for its next frantic shake up. Over the years the idea of using a plastic bottle with different contents developed into the creation of the 'Visi-bottle'. Perhaps it is the feeling of movement and weight as the water sloshes about inside, or maybe it is the gentle and controllable rearrangement of the contents that gives it child appeal. Even children for whom other toys seem to hold little interest sometimes respond to this type of toy. For very little effort, and no expense, it can certainly make a useful addition to a collection of toys to watch.

A Visi-bottle to Shake

Very quick

Do you remember the 'snowstorm' toys that were popular a few years ago? They can still be found occasionally in gift shops. A water-filled dome of clear plastic covers a tiny winter scene. Turn the toy upside down, then right way up and 'snowflakes' gently flutter through the water to settle over the scene.

A cheap and cheerful variation of this toy can be made in a jiffy. Fill a clear plastic bottle with water, sprinkle in a small amount of desiccated coconut or some oats and tightly screw on the cap. Give the bottle a quick shake to stir up the contents, and then watch the particles slowly sink to the bottom. The water tends to become cloudy eventually, but by then the toy will probably have lost its appeal!

An improved version can be made by filling a small clear plastic bottle with glycerine (from the chemist) and using silver glitter for the snow. These materials are more expensive, but may be worth it. The bottle can make an attractive ephemeral toy, perhaps for a 'frail' child who needs a low-effort plaything.

A Swishing Jar

Very quick

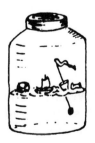

I first made this toy for a lively three-year-old who had both a hearing and a sight impairment. He was a 'wanderer'. It was difficult to persuade him to sit at the table and play with a toy even for a brief spell. Most playthings soon ended up on the floor. Not so the Swishing Jar! It was *large* and *heavy* and quite different from all the normal brightly coloured plastic toys he was usually offered. He would sit with his nose nearly touching the jar as he rocked it and watched the floating objects bob about on the surface of the water. When he was tired of looking at the ping-pong ball, corks and cotton reel, they could be exchanged for a tiny boat, some chips of polystyrene packaging or any other flotsam that happened to be to hand.

You can see from the illustration that the Swishing Jar is a converted sweet jar—the kind that, a few years ago might be thrown away by the owner of the sweet shop on the corner. They are still occasionally available from this source, but these days you may have to buy a plastic storage jar. If you make this toy for a child whose hands are large enough to unscrew the top, fix it in place with U-Hu or other plastic glue. This will avoid unwanted spillage but, of course, the contents of the bottle cannot be changed.

Divers in a Bottle

Quick

Daniel Hart,
Student on
Work Experience

I met Daniel when he was working in a Special Class for teenagers with severe learning difficulties. It was a wet day so, at playtime, the pupils were confined to the classroom. Daniel produced his water-filled bottle, complete with two divers, and began to play with it. As he squeezed the sides of the plastic bottle, the divers sank gracefully to the bottom. When he stopped squeezing, they bobbed up to the top again. He soon attracted a small group of children, all eager to have a go. For one girl, the fascination of this toy lasted the whole of playtime. She watched her friends play and when their interest waned, she seized the bottle. She soon discovered how to make the divers plummet to the bottom. Then she began to experiment by placing her hands on different parts of the bottle and applying more, or less, pressure to see how the divers would react.

Materials
- Plastic bottle with cap (e.g. fruit squash bottle).
- Two empty ink cartridges for the divers.
- A small lump of plasticine or Blu-tack.
- Water.

Method
Cut off the pricked ends of the cartridges. Wash them out. Seal the open ends with a blob of plasticine. *Fill* the bottle with water. Insert the divers. Replace the cap.

Note
When I copied this excellent toy, I found the amount of plasticine used was critical. Be too generous, and your divers will plunge straight to the bottom. Nothing for it but to empty out all the water and start again! If you do not add enough plasticine, no amount of squeezing will induce the divers to perform. This is why this toy is classified as 'Quick', rather than 'Instant'. Allow a little time for scientific experimentation!

LEARNING TO TRACK

Bubbles

Blowing bubbles is one of the sure-fire play successes of early childhood. They are mostly blown for the sheer pleasure of it but, if justification is needed for this indulgence, it can be said that watching bubbles makes a perfect 'tracking' activity. They float *slowly* in the direction of the air current and are full of entrancing colours. There is always the fun of trying to blow a huge one that will drift further than all the others before it ends in an unpredictable 'pop'.

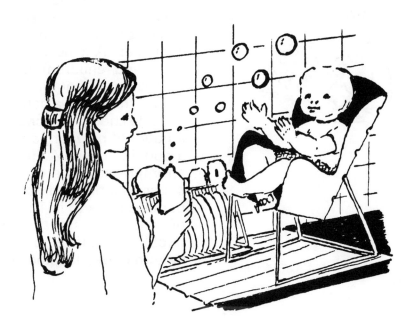

**More Spectacular
Bubbles and What to
Do with Them**

1. *Blowing a mound of bubbles*

Some children will have already discovered how to do this when they have vigorously blown through a straw into their beaker of milk— and probably been scolded for their bad manners!

Sometimes the art of 'bubbling' has to be learnt. When a straw is placed in her mouth, a child may think she is being offered a pleasant drink, and will suck instead of blow. What an unpleasant shock to end up with a mouthful of soapy water! One way to make sure this does not happen is to use a transparent drinking straw, or better still, a length of thin polythene tubing used in wine making. This can quickly be removed from the child's mouth if the liquid is seen to travel upwards.

Once having learnt to bubble efficiently, the obvious place for all this frothy activity is in the bath. At other times, a lot of mess can be avoided by putting the basin of bubble mixture inside a washing-up bowl or on a tray covered with a towel. This way the bubbles can pile up and spill over the edge of the basin, but the child and her surroundings should remain dry.

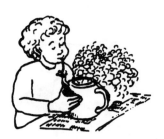

When the excitement of blowing bubbles in a basin begins to pall, try using an unusual container. A teacher at the Sense Centre (for deaf/blind children) puts bubble mixture in a teapot. Try it! Another use for a pile of bubbles is to turn them into a pattern. In the nursery class at a local school, I watched the teacher add a small amount of powder paint to the bubble mixture in a pudding basin. A little group of children raised an impressive pile of tinted bubbles. A sheet of paper was pressed gently on the top until some bubbles stuck to it. The paper was carefully lifted off and put aside to dry. We all watched the bubbles gradually pop, leaving behind a delicate pattern of overlapping circles.

2. *Blowing bubbles a different way*

One bath night my children discovered that a cotton reel (floating around as a bath toy!) made a good bubble pipe. A bubble could be blown by rubbing one end over the soap until a membrane formed, and directing a gentle stream of breath through the other. The cotton reel works just as well with bubble mixture, but it is wise to point the reel downwards to avoid the detergent trickling down the hole into the child's mouth.

An Elegant Bubble-blowing Toy

Long-lasting

Jo Sweeney,
Hospital Play Specialist

Jo visited a Science Workshop in the USA where she watched children raising mounds of bubbles by this simple method. The top of a yoghurt pot was covered with a circle of terry towelling which was held in place by a rubber band. A small hole was made in the side of the pot and a drinking straw inserted. After dipping the terry towelling top in bubble mixture, a child could blow through the straw. The more powerful his puff, the higher the mound of bubbles he could raise! Jo adapted this idea to make a robust toy.

Materials
- A plastic cup from a set of stacking cups with a diameter of at least 5cm (2″). The smaller the cup, the easier it is to build up enough pressure inside to raise the bubbles, so avoid the largest cups in the set.
- Terry towelling—an old face flannel will do.
- Shirring elastic—the thin, round kind used for gathering.
- Pony-tail hairband—a small elasticated ring of soft fabric.
- A drinking straw.
- A drill bit slightly larger than the drinking straw.
- Bubble mixture, *see below*.

Method
Cut a circle of terry towelling to cover the top of the stacking cup and reach about half way down the side. Keep it in place with the pony-tail band, and

trim off any excess terry towelling. Thread a needle with shirring elastic and sew the pony-tail hairband to the terry towelling with about two rows of running stitch. With the drill bit, make a hole in the side of the stacking cup, just below the pony-tail band. Dip the terry towelling *top* in bubble mixture. Insert a drinking straw in the hole and *blow*!

Note
If the bubble-blowing toy is to be used on another occasion by a different child, it is a simple matter to wash the terry towelling cap and insert a new drinking straw.

Recipe for Bubble Mixture

20 fl oz water
1 fl oz concentrated washing-up liquid
2 tablespoons glycerine (from the chemist)

Put all this in a plastic squash bottle and use as required.

A Visi-tube

Quick

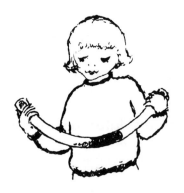

I invented this plaything when working as a toymaker in a school for children with severe learning difficulties. One of the teachers had requested a toy to help a particular boy. This lad had difficulty in holding an object with both hands, and usually opted out by only using his 'good' one. The more often he was able to solve his problems this way, the less likely he was to be able to make use of his 'lazy' hand. My first Visi-tube was an attempt to help him use both together. It would only work if held that way. It consisted of about 1m (40") of tough, clear, thick plastic tubing as used in home wine-making. One end of the tube was blocked off by ramming a cork well inside the rim, so that the only way of removing it would be with a corkscrew. Brightly coloured beads, tiny buttons etc., small enough to slide easily along the tube without getting jammed, were fed into the open end of the tube. Then this was corked up. The idea was to hold the tube at both ends, then tilt it by alternately raising and lowering each hand, so making the contents in the tube race from one end to the other and back again. The boy managed to make the beads move a little at the first try and was motivated gradually to improve his skill.

In the class was another boy who was reluctant to hold anything at all. After watching his friend play, he consented to hold one end of the Visi-tube while his teacher held the other. He cottoned on to the idea of rolling the beads from his end to hers by raising his arm, but it took some time for him to realise he must lower it to make them roll back again.

The rest of the class soon wanted to play too, and queued up to take turns. We encouraged more concentrated looking by masking off a section of the tube with opaque sticky tape. The boys learnt how to control the tube so that the contents could be hidden behind the tape.

I have since made slightly shorter Visi-tubes for a few of our toy library members. Emma, a four-year-old who also had difficulty in using both hands, had extra fun with hers. She was an articulate little girl and together we made up little stories to help her to control the tube. Perhaps the beads represented a train that must stop in the station—the masked off section of the tube. The passengers were cross if some of the carriages were left outside and they couldn't alight! Maybe the beads were 'children' out for a leisurely walk when all of a sudden the rain fell down and they must scuttle for shelter behind the tape. Sometimes the beads were tipped beyond the shelter and the children got wet. (Giggles from Emma!)

This toy is virtually indestructible and therefore can be suitable for 'tough guys'. It is not for use by an unsupervised rumbustious group. It might be swung about by one end and used as a weapon!

A Helicopter

Instant

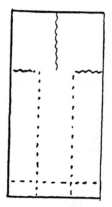

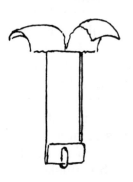

You need a rectangle of paper, say cheap notepaper, not too thick, about 10 × 20cm (4 × 8"). About a third of the way down one side, make a tear a third of the distance across and fold in the longer section. Repeat the process on the other side. (Your paper now vaguely resembles a garden spade!) Turn up the bottom and crease across firmly. A paper clip will keep it in place and add a little weight. To make the 'rotor blades', tear down from the middle of the top edge as far as the folded part. Bend one blade towards you and the other away from you. Give them both a slight curve as in the illustration. Now for the maiden flight! Hold the helicopter up high, let go, and watch it spiral its way towards the floor—in the manner of a sycamore seed.

Note
Watch which way your helicopter turns—clockwise or anti-clockwise? Bend the rotor blades in the opposite direction, and now see what happens!

A See-Saw Marble Run

Long-lasting

This is a 'general purpose' toy. It appeals to eyes, ears and hands. Children of many ages will spend a considerable time tipping the see-saw from one side to the other for the pleasure of watching—and listening to—the marbles as they scuttle down the central track. As with all see-saws, it works with a simple balancing action. The track, covered with perspex, curves in a gentle wavy line and the marbles travel from one end to the other, their speed varying according to the tilt of the see-saw. Once children understand the principle, they like to tip the see-saw very gradually to make the marbles travel at a snail's pace. (Make them go too slowly, and some will separate from the pack and roll back to base.)

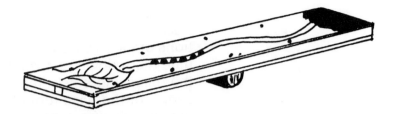

Michael Wason adapted this toy to represent a creepy crawly caterpillar. One end of the perspex was painted brown—to represent the earth—and on the other was painted a leaf. The marbles could shelter under the 'earth', then scuttle down the track to eat the 'leaf'—and back again, ad infinitum.

Note

Perspex is expensive. For a cheaper version for an individual child of known habits, try using thick industrial polythene, or, *if safe*, dispense with the cover altogether. Just issue the marbles at play time and collect them all up afterwards.

Materials
- About ten marbles. Small ones will do.
- One strip of plywood, about ¾ metre long, and thicker than the diameter of the marbles.
- Another strip of plywood, the same length, but slightly wider. It is for the base, so can be thinner.
- A block of wood, for the centre balancing point of the see-saw—say 7½ cm (3") × 10–12cm (4–4¾").
- A strip of perspex, the same size as the plywood base, to cover the top and keep the marbles in place.
- Some screws, paint, masking tape, wood glue.

Method

Cut the thick ply into two pieces with a gentle wavy line down the middle—a band saw does this job well. Do not make the curves too pronounced or the marbles will not run smoothly. With masking tape, temporarily fix one half of the see-saw track to the ply base. Leave a narrow gap, just wide enough to take the marbles comfortably, then tape the other half of the see-saw track to the base. When you are quite sure the marbles are running up and down the track with the maximum efficiency, mark the positions of the two halves of the see-saw track, but don't glue them down just yet. Next, round off the base of the balancing block. Temporarily fix the block to the centre of the base (double-sided Sellotape?) and try out the tilt of the see-saw. If this is too steep, the marbles will rush too quickly from one end to the other, and the block will need to be made a little lower. When you are satisfied all is well, glue the block to the base. Countersink, say, four screws through the base and into the block for extra strength. Sandpaper the sides of the track and the top of the base where the marbles will roll. Temporarily fix the two halves of the track to their lines on the base. Test again that the marbles will run freely. If so, screw and glue the sides to the base. Make small plugs of plywood for each end of the track to prevent the marbles from escaping. Sandpaper all the surfaces and paint them. When the paint is thoroughly dry, insert the marbles and cover the top with perspex. Fix it in place with plenty of screws.

Little Tumbling Men

Quick

This is a traditional toy sometimes found at craft markets or gift shops. It is a superb tracking toy, and the sight of the little man somersaulting down a slope never fails to excite both children and the adults caring for them.

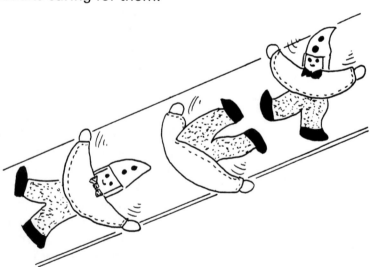

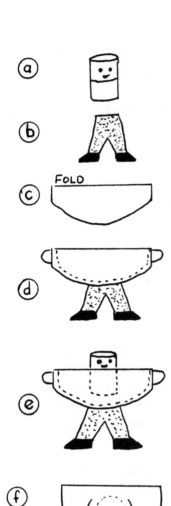

(a)

(b)

(c) FOLD

(d)

(e)

(f)

(g)

(h)

Many people have asked me for the pattern, so here goes ...

Materials
- A plastic film carton.
- A tool for removing the bottom and rim—small hack saw, or craft knife.
- A marble—as large as possible, but it must fit *easily* inside the carton.
- Scraps of felt—bright colours, with perhaps a little black for contrast.
- PVA adhesive.
- Needle and cotton.

Method
Cut off the rim and bottom of the film carton, converting it into a tube. For the face, cut off a small strip of felt (pink or brown), long enough to cover about half the tube, and wide enough to wrap completely round it. Make the features—embroider them or use tiny felt circles stitched on. Stick the face to the tube, as in illustration (a). While the adhesive is drying, cut out the legs and feet in single felt (b). Shoes are an optional extra. Cut out the jacket from folded felt (c). Cut out two small hands and pin them to the ends of the arms. Pin the legs in position. Stab stitch all these pieces to the jacket (d). Cut a slit in the top centre of the jacket, just large enough to take the tube. Smear the bottom half of the tube fairly liberally with adhesive and insert it into the jacket. Press the two together and hold them in position to give the adhesive a chance to stick (e). Cut out the head piece as in the illustration (f). It must be able to cover the top of the tube and overlap the forehead, back and sides of the tube. *Put in the marble!* Now cover the top of the tube with the head piece (g). It sometimes needs a bit of jiggery pokery to make it fit. I find it best to spread adhesive on the man's forehead, then round the back and sides of his head, and temporarily bind the head piece in place with cotton. This holds the felt surfaces together while the adhesive sets. Cut out the hat in single felt (h). Sew felt spots or sequins to it. (If you only stick them on they

will not survive many tumbles.) Remove the cotton binding from the head. Stick the hat to the front of the head piece (i), and again bind it with cotton until the adhesive sets. Neaten the join between the face and the jacket by stitching on a felt collar or a bow tie.

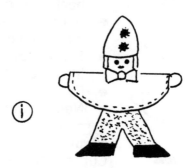

Of course, the little tumbling man needs a sloping surface for his acrobatics. A piece of board covered with felt and propped up on a few books works well; so does an ironing board, closed flat, covered with a blanket and inclined, to make the required slope.

Note
It is possible for a child to tear the felt and get at the marble inside. This toy must only be used under adult supervision.

LEARNING TO SCAN

The Game of Peep-Bo

This old favourite has been enjoyed by babies since time immemorial. It is the element of anticipation and surprise that they find so delightful. A face, or a teddy, that pops up from behind the back of the arm chair—sometimes over the top, sometimes round the side—is sure to appeal to the baby's sense of humour. Played with sensitivity so that the surprise object is always within the child's range of vision, this simple game can provide plenty of practise in scanning, (searching).

A Peep-bo Puppet

Almost Instant

Mme Schneider

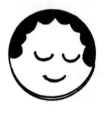

Mme Schneider lives in Switzerland and is a teacher of visually impaired children. She finds this 'high contrast' little puppet ideal for a quick game of Peep-bo. She claims it is made in a jiffy, and she is right!

Cut two circles of white material, about the size of a saucer. Stitch or stick them together for just over half way round, leaving an opening at the bottom for your hand. Slip some stiff paper (or card) between the circles to prevent the ink from spreading through, and draw a face on both sides with a black marker pen. Perhaps one face could be happy and the other sad, or one awake and the other asleep. Draw some black hair round the top of the face. Remove the paper, put your hand inside, and show the puppet to your child. Now you are ready for a game of Peep-bo. Make the little face pop out from behind the curtain, or suddenly appear over the top of the arm chair.

Scrapbooks

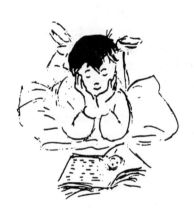

These can be very personal possessions when made for a particular child, and can often hold his attention when all other books fail. If you have not yet made a scrapbook, you may find the following hints helpful.

1. *Make the subject of your book topical*
   Children are primarily interested in everything that directly concerns themselves, and a book entitled 'Me' can be a winner! The pages could include photos of the child and his family, and pictures of his favourite toys, his chosen make of car, pets, favourite food, picture postcards, tickets saved from an outing,—even the wrapping from a bar of chocolate can have special significance.

2. *Keep the book short*
   A child who is just old enough to enjoy a scrapbook is likely to have a limited span of attention, and may still be at the tearing stage. It is better to spend the time making four thin books than one magnificent fat one. This way the books can have more variety and, should the temptation to tear

become overwhelming, it is not as disastrous as the destruction of a large book would be.

3. *Use the strongest and most colourful materials*
   Plain wallpaper (not the bumpy kind or vinyl coated, or the scraps will not stick properly) can be pasted onto card from cartons, cereal packets, washing powder boxes, etc., to make the pages of a board book. These pages can be tied together loosely in three places so that they will turn over easily. Pages can also be cut from thick brown paper and stitched together. Coloured sticky tape can be used to reinforce the edges, and this will also cheer up the brown paper.

4. *Make sure the edges of the scraps are well stuck down* or the temptation to 'pick' will be irresistible!

Note
If you have taken the trouble to make a special scrapbook, it will be disappointing if it is soon torn. Look at it during a quiet moment when you can talk about the pictures and savour them together. The book could be a firm favourite and subject to heavy wear. It may be worthwhile protecting the pages with clear sticky-backed plastic (from a large stationer's shop). A special scrapbook that has taken time and effort to make may well become a family treasure and be worth preserving.

A Scrap Sheet

Instant

This is just a large sheet of paper fixed to the wall or the back of a door. It must be at the right height for the child to see properly, and to be able to point to the pictures. Every day a new one can be added until there is no more room.

A Zigzag Scrapbook

Quick

This makes a change from the conventional scrapbook, and can be made to stand up so that the child can see all the pictures in a long line. Stiff paper or thin card is folded zigzag fashion so that it can close up and open out like a concertina. Pictures can be stuck to both sides. A good subject for this kind of book might be 'In the Street'. Pictures of cars, lorries, a fire engine, an ambulance, a bus, a removal van, bicycles, people, etc. could be pasted on each section of the book. When opened out, it will show a long picture like a frieze.

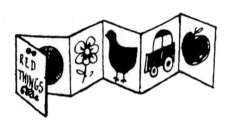

Rag Books

Long-lasting

Rag books for young children have undoubted advantages over paper ones. The pages are thick and easy to turn. They are virtually untearable and can be dribbled on—even chewed—and then restored to their first glory by a quick swirl in the washing machine.

If your child is at the rag book stage, but is not attracted by commercial ones, this may be because the pictures are too small for him to see properly, or are cluttered up with words, or are just not about things that interest him. Why not try making him a special one?

Materials
- Plain material for the pages. Unbleached calico is best. It is strong and cheap.
- Nursery curtaining for the pictures. This is usually printed in bold colours and has clear pictures which make excellent illustrations for a rag book. Search around fabric shops, market stalls, jumble sales and car boot sales (for second-hand curtains), and you will find a choice of animals, nursery rhymes, spacemen, cartoon characters and many more.
- A sewing machine.

Method

Decide on the size of your proposed book, then cut the plain material into pieces twice as wide as each page. Each strip will be doubled over, so that the fold makes the turning edge of the page. Cut out the pictures you have chosen, leaving a narrow border round the edge for the stitching. Using a very narrow machine stitch, attach two pictures to every piece of material, one each side of the fold. Change to a narrow zigzag stitch and sew round them all again. To make up the pages, put the pictures face to face, and straight stitch along the top and bottom of each page. You have now made a bag. The open side will become the spine of the book. Turn the bag inside out, so that the pictures now show. Press each page, and sew them all together at the open ends. They will probably be too thick to go under the machine. I join two or three by machine, then oversew them all with button thread. A strip of material sewn over the spine will cover the raw edges and make the book look neater.

If you enjoy sewing, it can be rewarding to make the pictures as a collage of your own design, perhaps incorporating a variety of textures. This kind of book makes a good present. It is washable, and well worth making for a toy library or hospital play scheme, where it can be enjoyed by a succession of children.

Picture Window Rag Books

Long-lasting

Every factory-made rag book is designed for babies. It is impossible to find one suitable for an older child with learning difficulties or hand function problems. The Picture Window Rag Book is unique, because it includes all the advantages of easily turned pages, indestructibility and washability (at a low temperature) *and* it can be made interesting for a child of any age—just like the family photograph album.

Each page is empty, except for a clear plastic window stitched down on three sides. The fourth side is left free so the photograph, picture postcard of any other pictures of the same size can be inserted between the page and the plastic window. By this simple method the pictures can be changed as often as necessary. One week, perhaps, the book will feature photos of the family and pets. These might be replaced by pictures of vehicles and street scenes, to be followed by photographic memories of a school trip.

I have made several of these books for individual children, each with special needs. One was for a girl of eleven. She could not walk without support and was unable to speak. She was also partially sighted. My aim was to try to widen the scope of her playtime by offering her an alternative to shaking various noisemakers or banging two toys together. Her book contained six pages. The pictures needed to be large so the windows were made 20 × 20cm (8 × 8"). They were stitched to the right hand pages only. I felt this would make it easier for her to learn to turn the pages over. I drew large, clear pictures of her toys and clothes, her family car and her wheelchair. I also made a few extra pages from black paper, and decorated them with diffraction stickers bought off the roll at a local toy shop. On a bright day, these showed up brilliantly in the sunlight and gave her particular pleasure.

Another book was made when my little friend Rupert was two years old. He had a skin problem, and his toys needed to be soft to avoid friction and, of course, they were washed frequently to keep them hygienic. His book contained ten pages, and there was a window on both sides. Each window measured 17 × 12cm (6¾ × 4¾"), the right size to hold a photograph or a picture postcard. His illustrations were of people he knew, and of parts of his village, plus some specially made ones to help him to recognise colours and to count. (A bunch of balloons and a collection of pairs of shoes, to name but two examples.)

If you decide to make a Picture Window Rag Book, first ask yourself how many pages it should have, and then what size the pictures should be. Then consult the 'shopping list' below.

Materials
- Fabric for the pages. Unbleached calico is best.
- Plastic material for the windows. I used PVC from the soft furnishing department of a large store.

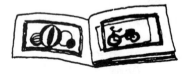

The plastic must be pliable, for it must accept machine stitching, and be able to bend when the pages are turned inside out.

- Black tape, or black bias binding for the frames.
- Plenty of pictures. Collect several sets the same size, so that they can be easily interchanged.

Method

Suppose your book is to have a picture on each page, as in the illustration. To make one page, cut a strip of calico twice as wide as the finished page size. Fold it in half, and crease it firmly down the fold. This will be the turning edge of the page. Open out the calico. The front and back of the page are now in line, (with the crease down the middle) ready to receive the windows.

Cut two windows from the PVC, making them about 1cm wider all round than the pictures they will cover. Make the frames from the tape. Cut it into lengths corresponding to the sides of the windows, allowing a little extra for tucking under at the corners. Position the tape on three sides of the window, so that about half overlaps the PVC. Sew it to the PVC with a single row of stitching. On the fourth side (the one that is to be left unattached to the page) bind the tape round the PVC and attach it with two rows of stitching. Now sew the frames to the page. Arrange for the open ends to face the spine. This will make it more difficult for the children to remove the pictures or for them to fall out accidentally. Pin the other three sides to the page and stitch them in position. Fold the front and back of the page together with the frames face to face. Stitch along the top and bottom edges, making a bag with the spine side open. Turn the bag right side out. Lightly press the *edges*. Avoid the PVC, of course, or you will melt it—and have a very messy iron to clean! Make as many similar pages as you want.

Make a front and back cover very slightly larger than the pages. There is a chance to embroider or applique a design here, or you can go for the easy option and use a pretty fabric. Join the pages and covers together in pairs, with the machine, then oversew the lot with button thread. Cover the spine with ribbon, a strip of fabric or braid, to hide the raw edges and the oversewing.

LOOKING AROUND

Some Instant Suggestions

The next time morale is low because rain bespatters the window pane, turn the raindrops into a looking game and have races between them! When the weather cheers up and you are indoors by a sunny window, why not play with Jack-a-dandies? These are the brilliant reflections made by sunlight bouncing off a shiny object, and can easily be made to 'dance' on the ceiling. Small, unbreakable mirrors make splendid Jack-a-dandies, but any shiny surface will do, even a bowl of water. (Slightly ruffle the surface to make changing, delicate patterns.) Perhaps, when you were at school you assumed an air of innocence as you reflected the sun off your knife and dazzled your friend! There is a knack in controlling a Jack-a-dandy—for a start, the shiny object must face the sun. To direct the reflection in a certain direction calls for considerable hand-eye coordination!

At night time, Torch Hee is a good game to play in the dark. Each player has a hand torch. One switches on and directs her beam over the walls and ceiling. The other player switches on and tries to impose her beam on the first one. When she succeeds, it is her turn to switch on first ... or just make up the rules as you go along.

A Seeing Saunter

This is the kind of walk when time is of no consequence. So often this is not the case. Time presses and the ground must be covered as quickly as possible. Not so on a 'seeing saunter'. The distance covered may only be to the end of the street but, on the way, there will have been time to examine the patterns on the drain covers, notice the designs in the brickwork of the houses, admire the gardens, find plants growing in unlikely places, read the numbers on the gates, even perhaps find some adventurous insects also out for a stroll. Whatever the child's environment may be, town, country or in between, for those who look, there are always fresh things to discover.

A String Ring

Adopt a scientific sampling technique. Make a 'string ring' and you have an unusual way of focusing your child's attention on one tiny patch of the world that surrounds him. Imagine you are both sitting on the grass. All you have to do is to mark out a small area with a circle of string and peer intently into it! Soon both of you will notice not only the grass with its many shades of green, but also the plants and mosses, all contributing to the greenery. Look carefully, and you might see a worm throwing up a cast, or a tiny insect struggling through the jungle of leaves. Because the area under scrutiny is defined by the string ring, your child is less likely to be distracted by the wider view and some concentrated observation should result. What a pleasant way of 'learning to look'.

Shopping Search

Try this searching activity when next you visit the supermarket.

Susan's Mum invented 'Shopping Search'. Susan was a profoundly deaf little girl. Her mother was always looking for an opportunity to enlarge her vocabulary and help her associate words with objects. She made a collection of pictures of food. She found these in magazines, or on the tins and packets in her store cupboard. Each picture was mounted on card (possibly the backs of old Christmas cards), and the name of each item was written under its picture. Before each shopping expedition, she would show her shopping list to Susan, who would then match the word on the list to the one under the picture. All the necessary pictures were taken to the supermarket, where Susan could search for the real thing among the shelves. This game is a winner. It can turn a sometimes stressful shopping expedition into an enjoyable experience packed full of learning! It is especially recommended for children with speech problems, slow learners, and the busy ones!

GAMES FOR OLDER CHILDREN

These games are best played with a patient adult who is prepared to wait. Given *time*, most children with some degree of sight love to play tabletop games such as Ludo or Snakes and Ladders. If shared with their peer group, problems may occur. Sighted children may take their own turn too quickly, or even play *for* the child with a sight problem. With the best of intentions, they may shake the dice for him or even move his pieces on the board. Either way, the sighted child is reducing our child's self-confidence and robbing him of the chance to make his own decisions ... and practise his scanning!

Kim's Game

Instant

This is a game requiring keen observation and a good memory. It can easily be adapted to meet the needs of children of varying ages and abilities. It is usually played as a group game, but works just as well with one child and an adult.

The Basic Game
Arrange some easily recognisable objects on a tray, e.g. a matchbox, cotton reel, thimble, button, pencil, etc. The number of the objects chosen will depend on the ability of the child. He then has time to look at all the objects, and memorise their position on the tray. He hides his eyes while one object is removed. When he opens them, he has another look at the tray and guesses which object is missing. Then it is his turn to remove an object for you to identify.

Variations
Instead of taking an object away, another can be added to the tray, or the position of two objects can be interchanged. Sometimes the child can help to collect the items for the tray, perhaps choosing only round shapes, or rectangular ones, or those of a certain colour. Because he has contributed to the collection, a child with a poor memory will have a better chance of identifying them.

Tabletop matching games

When a child can pick out two identical pictures from a pile of jumbled-up pairs, she is ready to move on to one of the simpler games of picture-matching dominoes and lottos. These games call for accurate observation and an ability to wait your turn. They are also an excellent way of reinforcing the meaning of known words, and adding new ones to a child's vocabulary.

Dominoes

There are plenty of domino games in the toy shops, but they are so easy to make at home, and can be produced in so many ways, that it seems a shame not to have a go! Homemade ones can add variety to the commercial ones and, perhaps, make the game possible for children who cannot manage those on sale. For some ideas you will find Tactile Dominoes on (p. 115), Button Dominoes (p. 116) and some more made specially for children with a visual handicap on (p. 117). To make your own set of dominoes, cut out rectangles of card of a suitable size to take two pictures. Leave the first half of one rectangle blank, then add one of the pictures of a pair. Start the next rectangle with the twin picture, and finish it with the first picture of the next pair. Complete the set in this way. The last rectangle will end with a blank.

Diffraction Sticker Dominoes

Long-lasting

Diffraction stickers are small, brightly-coloured pictures of objects or patterns that catch the light. For maximum effect, the stickers need to be mounted on a matt black background and played with under a bright light (sunlight or artificial). The effect can be sensational!

Diffraction stickers are sold off the roll, or in packs, at large stationers, toy and gift shops, and sometimes at the little shop on the corner. You may need to visit several shops to collect a sufficient variety of pairs of stickers.

Materials
- Pairs of diffraction stickers, *at least* eight.

- Rectangles of thick card, one for each pair of stickers and one extra. Suggested size 12cm × 6cm (5" × 2½").
- If black card is not easily available, paint what you have with black acrylic paint, or cover the rectangles with polyurethane adhesive and black poster paper.

Method

Lay the rectangles end to end in a long line. Arrange your pairs of stickers in a pleasing sequence. Leave the left hand half of the first rectangle blank, then apply the stickers domino fashion. (Right half of one rectangle matches the left half of the following one.) End with a blank.

If you want a more complicated game with many pieces, use a sheet of diffraction paper from Eduplay (p. 4), large stationers, art shops, etc. and cut out geometric shapes. It is worthwhile investing in a plastic geometric template which you can buy from any large stationers. This ensures that the shapes really do match and saves a lot of fiddling about with compasses and set squares.

Footnote

I showed a set of these dominoes to a group of teachers. One was delighted with the idea and promptly gave it an original twist. She said her Great Aunt had sight problems and would dearly like to play games with her young children. A set of these dominoes would make that possible—and everybody would be happy!

Picture Lottos

Lotto games consist of a set of base boards with pictures printed on them, and another set of the same pictures printed on small cards which, in play, are matched to those on the base boards. Usually all the little cards are shuffled up, then placed in a pile in the middle of the table. The children take it in turns to turn up the top picture. If they need it for their base board, they keep it. If not, it is returned to the bottom of the pile. The game takes quite a long time to play by this method. For young children, or those with a short attention span, I change the rules a little! Everyone has a base board, but the method of distributing the small cards can vary according to the needs of the children playing. Perhaps they have very little, or no, speech, yet know the names of many objects. A leader who has no difficulty with words is appointed. (This is usually an adult.) The leader turns up the first card, says the name of the object on it and, if nobody recognises the word, shows the picture to the children. The one who needs it, claims it, and places it on top of the corresponding picture on her base board. The game continues until all the pictures on every base board are covered.

Young children with verbal ability like to play the following way. The base boards are distributed and the small cards placed in the centre. One child picks a card, keeps the picture secret, but names the object on the card. The child who needs it, claims it. Taking turns in rotation, the next child turns up a card and, if lucky, it may be a picture she wants, so she can keep it. If not, she must give it away. If the game is played competitively, the child owning the first complete base board is the winner. Bingo!

Bought Lottos may not be suitable for young children with learning difficulties. The pictures are often too complicated, the pieces too numerous, and the time it takes to finish the game is likely to be too long for children with a short attention span. By the time they are mature enough to manage bought lottos, the pictures may be uninteresting to them and unsuitable for their age. The solution to all these problems is to make your own—a tailormade version.

A First Lotto

Long-lasting

This simple game is really just picture matching made into a group activity, but it helps children to understand the new idea of matching the pictures to a base board and, as it is a group game, they have to wait for their turn. It is patently clear when they match the pictures correctly, and the eyes of every child will be following the matching process to make sure each player gets it right!

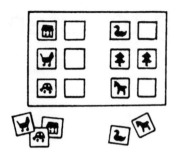

Materials

- Cardboard for the base boards and matching cards. (I used the fronts and backs of soap powder packets for my first set.)
- Pictures. Draw these yourself, (tracing off the second picture to make sure it matches) or use templates, or cut suitable pictures from gift wrapping paper, or buy a pack of Picture Identification Labels from NES Arnold, p. 4.
- PVA adhesive, craft knife and metal ruler for cutting the cardboard.
- Clear sticky-backed plastic for protecting the finished cards. (From large stationers or educational suppliers.)
- A container for all the pieces.

Method

First collect the pictures. The Picture Identification Labels mentioned above save a lot of effort and give a professional-looking result. They have an adhesive backing dispensing with the need for PVA adhesive. The size and number of pictures on the base board will, of course, determine its dimensions. Look at the illustration and arrange your pairs of pictures the same way. You may need more, or longer columns for your game. Rule up your base board in columns of pairs of squares (or rectangles) leaving a gap between each column. Stick one picture from each pair onto the base board. Stick the other to the small card which will, in play, be placed next to its partner on the base board. Wait until the adhesive is thoroughly dry, then cover all the pieces with clear sticky-backed plastic.

Learning to listen

THINKING BACK TO MY 'PAPER BAG EXPERIMENT' described on p. 5, when I temporarily deprived myself of the ability to see, I am sure my ears as well as my fingers were working overtime. It is obvious that when one of our senses is less than perfect, it pays dividends to compensate for the deficiency by developing the other senses as fully as possible. A child who learns about sounds as part of her play will unwittingly be developing her listening skills and expanding her aural memory. This will help her to identify and sort out the jumble of noises that daily surround us. As a little exercise in listening, take a pencil and paper and time yourself for five minutes by the clock. In that brief time write down all the sounds you hear. I live in a quiet cul-de- sac, but even so, as I write I am aware of the slight hum from the central heating (just now receiving a boost), foot-steps and voices in the street, my neighbour closing a door, a van passing ... and so it goes on. A child who has only been in this world for a short time must learn to make sense of all the sounds which surround her, and build up a memory bank. Sounds, if they can't be experienced at first hand, need to be explained. When they are familiar to us, it can be so easy to forget to describe them as they happen—the aeroplane passing overhead or the approach of the milkman with his clinking bottles ...

When we think about toys with an inbuilt sound, rattles (a baby's first real toy) are sure to come to mind. These wonderful playthings have their origins rooted in ancient history. (I have read that there is an Egyptian rattle in a museum dating from hundreds of years BC.) They have certainly stood the test of time. One of the great delights of a rattle is that the sound it makes is in the control of the child. It responds to her shaking, but when she drops it or keeps it still, there is silence ... a first lesson in cause and effect!

All the noisemakers in this chapter need human intervention—yours, or the child's—to activate them. This gives a choice between sound and silence. If a child is surrounded by noises, it can be difficult for her to pick out a particular one. The situation can be similar to a lively party where we find it nearly impossible to make ourselves heard above the general hubbub and background music. Moral—if you are aiming to develop a child's listening skills, exclude extraneous sounds as much as possible, introduce new sounds gradually, and don't forget to include some soft ones!

NOISY MOBILES

Dancing Danglement

Quick

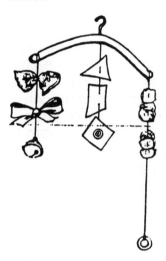

A Bamboo Mobile

Long-lasting

This is a mobile that does not rely on a draught to make it move. It is activated by 'baby power'. When the string is pulled, the mobile will bob about and set all the noisemakers jangling.

A coat-hanger is hung out of reach of the child, but where he can see it easily. An assortment of noisy objects and some colourful ones are tied to the hanger. These might include a bunch of bells, a string of foil milk bottle tops, a rattle, a tassel of brightly-coloured ribbons, cellophane sweet wrappers—tied in the middle to make them look like butterflies ... Make about three strings of these with one considerably longer than the others. This is the one for the child to pull. Make it easy to hold by tying a ring or cotton reel to the end. Be sure the strings cannot slip off the hanger—either drill holes for them or cut notches in the top. On a plastic hanger, bind the strings in place with Sellotape.

This mobile can be used in two ways: in version 1, the mobile is hung out of reach (like the Dancing Danglement above), and the child pulls a string to make the sound; in version 2, as shown, it is hung within reach for a 'hands on' experience. In this case, the child can run his hands along the line of bamboo tubes to make them strike together. This mobile is weather resistant, so is suitable for hanging outside—on a verandah perhaps, or in the winter from the branches of a bare tree, where it could provide a welcome spot of colour in a dreary winter landscape.

Materials

- A length of broomstick or thick dowel for support.
- Bamboo garden canes … say two.
- An old knitting needle.
- Paint. Acrylic is best, but poster will do.
- Polyurethane varnish.
- Thin nylon cord for suspending the support.
- Strong, thin thread for hanging the bamboo sections.
- Beads—optional, but they make the bamboo sections hang better and look pretty.
- Tools—a small saw, two drills, a craft knife, sandpaper.

Method

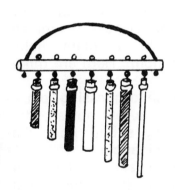

Divide the bamboo canes into separate sections by cutting about 10mm (¼") above each joint. The sections will be different lengths and thicknesses. Discard any split or faulty ones and keep about eight to ten of the best. With a craft knife, scratch away all the waxy surface on the outside of each section. (Work away from yourself, and take care.) It is important to remove all the waxy surface or the paint will not stick properly and will chip off when the sections knock together. Rub each section with sandpaper to ensure that the surface is smooth and clean. Drill a small hole, just large enough to take the hanging thread, down through the joint at the top of each section. Remove the pith in the middle with a knitting needle. Hold the cane up to your eye and you should now be able to see right through it. Poke the hanging thread through the hole in the top of the section and out through the bottom. Tie a very large knot on the end, or better still, thread it through a small bead to prevent it from pulling out through the hole in the joint. Paint all the bamboo sections in bright colours, and when they are dry, protect each with at least two coats of polyurethane varnish. Decide how you would like them to hang and arrange them in a row. Leave a gap between each— about the width of a section—and measure the space they occupy. Cut the broomstick (or dowel) hanger about 8cm (3") longer. Drill holes at appropriate intervals along it, one for each section of bamboo and one each end for the suspending cord. Tie each section to the hanger. If you use beads, thread one as a spacer between a section and the hanger, and perhaps one on the top (as in the illustration) to make sure the section will not drop off. Finally, attach the suspending cord and a pull string if you are making version 1.

A Circular Mobile a Child Can Sit Inside

Quick

Like the two mobiles above, this one also rewards a child for making an effort! In this case, he sits surrounded by potential noisemakers which seem to invite him to give them a biff.

The hanger for this mobile is a large plastic hoop. It must be suspended horizontally from three or four points, and hung at the correct height to encircle the child's head like a giant halo. Noisemakers dangle from the hoop. Here are three suggestions.

- Use balloons. To keep the child guessing, put a few grains of rice inside some, but not all. The rice will make a soft rustling sound. Keep the strings fairly short or they will tangle.
- Copy the mobile made by a teacher at Linden Bennet School. Cardboard rolls (from baking foil or paper towels) were painted in bright colours or covered with foil paper. A bell was hung inside some of them.
- At White Lodge Centre, Margaret Gillman bedizened her hoop with tin lids. (No sharp edges!) The spacing was important. Hitting one lid should make it swing against its neighbours.

MAKING OPPORTUNITIES FOR ATTENTIVE LISTENING

For young children

Consider the neighbours, and the rest of the family, but when the time is right, look around the kitchen

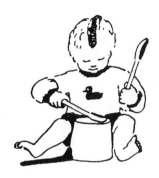

for some 'instant' percussion instruments. A wooden spoon and an upturned saucepan or biscuit tin will make a perfect drum. Two tough plastic egg cups can be banged together to make a noise like castanets, and an old spoon stirred round a wire sieve will make a gentle whirring sound ... The child is sure to invent her own sounds. A three-year-old of my acquaintance illustrates this point. She had nearly finished eating her yoghurt. In her efforts to scrape up every bit, she was running her spoon round the bottom of the pot. This had ridges, like the spokes of a wheel. She found that drawing her spoon over these made a loud and distinctive sound quite capable of stopping the meal-time conversation.

Use a particular sound to anticipate a certain activity. In Victorian families a gong would summon everyone to the meal. In modern times, the Ship's Bell Rattle (p. 59) might serve the same purpose. Even a simple action such as splashing your hand in the water before putting a child in the bath, will give him a sound clue of what is about to happen.

If you can remember to say 'Up you come' every time before picking baby up, the frequent repetition will help him to recognise the 'tune' of the phrase long before he can understand the words. The daily routine can be full of such noisy little incidents, and each will help a child to be more aware of his surroundings and add to his sense of security.

Speak and sing to your child as much as you can. Describe your actions as you care for him and go about your work. All babies need to listen for many months before they are ready to try to make the sounds of speech. Some children with special needs may require a very long listening time before they can sort out all the sounds that surround them. If they do not appear to respond, or if they are 'good' and content to lie quietly until the next meal, it is so easy to forget to keep up the chatter! Nursery rhymes and finger plays and jingles for body awareness like 'This little piggy went to market' can come to the rescue!

A Trail of Noisy Objects

Instant

Pam Courtney,
Teacher

When children are constantly on the move, they are exercising both their muscles and their brains. As they explore their surroundings, they learn from all the new experiences and discoveries that come their way. A child with a visual handicap may need to be coaxed from the security of her own special corner, and the same reluctance to explore can also be a problem with those slow learners who seem perfectly happy to stay put. Without help, such children are unlikely to develop either physically or mentally as quickly as they should.

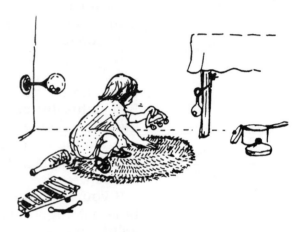

One way of increasing such a child's self-confidence and persuading her to 'have a go', might be to follow Pam's suggestion and lay a trail of noisy objects. Her intention is to lure the child from one noisemaker to the next, using anything that has child-appeal. The trail could include favourite sound-producing toys and rattles, the ever-popular saucepan and wooden spoon, or even an unfamiliar junk rattle like a few stones in a tin. At first, the child needs to be introduced to the idea of moving from one noisemaker to the next. Perhaps she starts by playing happily with a familiar rattle. When this begins to pall, her attention may be attracted by someone starting to play a xylophone softly, fairly close to her, but just out of reach. If she wants to know more about this fascinating new sound, she must move towards it (perhaps coaxed by some encouraging words). At a later stage, when she feels more confident, the trail of noisy objects can be laid in a line across the floor—or round the edge of the carpet—for her to discover in her own time. This activity will give her an idea of the layout of the room, and help her to find her way around.

For older children

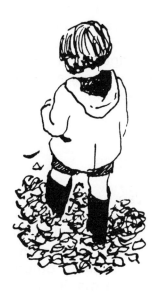

Try taking your child on a 'listening loiter'. Like the 'Seeing Saunter' on p. 43, the object of this particular walk is not to reach a destination, but to stop and listen at frequent intervals to all the sounds going on around. If you listen really hard, you will be surprised at the number you can identify in quite a short while. It is also fun for children to use the environment for making sounds—perhaps jumping on a drain cover, scuffing through the autumn leaves, dragging a stick along a wooden fence or across iron railings, blowing across a blade of grass held tightly between the thumbs—what a variety of sounds can be created by even these few activities.

Few homes are without radio or TV these days, but sometimes these facilities do little to encourage children to listen properly. The saying 'Familiarity breeds contempt' may very well apply here. The solution may be to use the *off* button more frequently, and when the *on* button is used, to give the programme proper attention. Treat yourself to a break from the chores. Sit down quietly and listen or watch together. Perhaps you can sing or dance to the music, discuss the plot, explain unusual words ... With your help, the child will be having a true listening experience.

Try making a sound picture. For this you need a cassette recorder and quite a lot of imagination. First think of a situation, then imagine all the noises that combine to make that situation recognisable. Imagine a walk down the High Street. If it is not pedestrianised, there will be the noises of the traffic, perhaps a Police car or an Ambulance in a hurry, footsteps on the pavement, scraps of conversations, maybe a barking dog or even a busker! Of course, all these sounds can be recorded in the street in the real situation. They can also be imitated by various means at home. A 'sound picture' was made in this way by a group of teenagers with learning difficulties. They first went for a walk by the river and, on returning to their classroom, they tried to recreate on tape the sounds they had heard. They used the Slither Box (p. 60) to indicate footsteps on the gravel tow-path. The sound of the wind in the reeds was made by rubbing the palms of their hands together. Someone dabbled his hand in a bowl of water to represent the lapping of the ripples against the bank and, of course, the siren of the tripper boat and the quacking of the ducks could not be left out.

HOMEMADE NOISEMAKERS

Here are some noisemakers that can be made from odds and ends. Their size and noisiness can easily be adapted, so there should be something suitable for every child, however special their need. Some of the noisemakers can be shaken with one hand, others encourage the use of two. Most can be manipulated by children who have restricted movements.

Making a noise is one of the universal pleasures of childhood. Being able to shake, rattle or bang on a drum can give more than just sensory pleasure. To be in control of the sound he makes can give a child a little more confidence in himself, and a lovely sense of power—especially if the sounds he makes produce a reaction in others. Think of the horrible noise of a knife scraping across a plate, and the way it sets our teeth on edge! The noisemakers suggested here are much more socially acceptable. Used purposefully, as in a band, or being played in time to the radio, these simple 'instruments' can help children to listen more carefully, and may even help to improve their coordination and powers of concentration.

A Rattle from a Fruit Juice Bottle

Instant

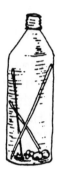

This rattle is ideal for a child who has just learnt to sit up, or for an older, gentle child. Its size, light weight and transparency give it child appeal. Its owner is likely to spend ages shaking the bottle, watching the contents bob about inside, and trying to make the loudest possible noise.

Wash the bottle thoroughly, and make sure it is really dry. If any moisture remains, it will form condensation, and the contents may stick together and not rattle properly. Practically any filling may be used but, in the interests of safety, it is best to stick to edible items like spaghetti, rice, lentils, etc. If you are certain the child will not manage to undo the lid, a few brightly-coloured buttons and some scraps of foil paper will look more attractive, and possibly make a louder noise. Once the contents are inside, the lid must be fixed on securely with polystyrene cement (e.g. U-Hu). Make sure this is set before offering the rattle to the child.

A Ship's Bell Rattle

Quick

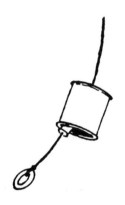

The special feature of this rattle is that it is capable of generating plenty of decibels! It can be either hand held, or tied to a suitable point such as a cot play bar or, for a child lying on the floor, the rung of a chair. When tied to something, it can make a useful rattle for children who tend to throw or drop their toys. I used the prototype, hand held, when I wanted to attract the attention of a group of children, and signal a change of activity.

Remove the lid from the tin and save it. It has a nicely turned lip—no sharp edges—and could come in handy for another toy! (e.g. the Sit Inside Mobile, p. 54) Wash the tin thoroughly and dry it. Punch a hole in the centre of the bottom. Push from the outside inwards so that the rough edges are inside. Thread about 45 cm (18") of string or piping cord through the hole. The latter is better—it looks more attractive and is soft to feel. Leave a tail of cord (for the clapper), then tie a large knot in the cord to prevent it from pulling out of the tin, and another knot outside—to keep the cord in place and stop it from disappearing inside. Make the clapper by threading a *large* wooden bead, or a cotton reel or a wooden brick with a hole drilled in it, onto the tail of cord. Tie a knot to prevent it from falling off. Make sure the clapper is in the right position to strike the tin, and produce the maximum noise. Tie a ring to the end of the tail to make it easier to grasp. Possibly, decorate the tin with Humbrol enamel.

A Tin Roller Rattle for the Floor

Quick

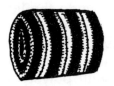

Here is another rattle made from a treacle tin (or similar.) It is particularly useful for a child who is just starting to crawl or bottom-shuffle, because its major feature is that it will not travel too fast or too far. Put some fish grit or a few small pebbles in the tin. Do not overload it or it will hardly roll at all! Hammer the lid on *firmly*. Make a fabric cover, (or crochet one,) which entirely covers the tin—two circles and a strip of the right size, firmly stitched together. The cover gives the tin a pleasant feel and makes it difficult for inquisitive fingers to remove the lid. When you lie the tin on its side, ready for play, give it a push. The grit will settle in the curved part touching the floor. This makes a distinctive noise and slows down the action nicely.

A Jumbo Shaker

Quick

Rosemary Hemmett, Toy Librarian

Do you ever search in vain for a really large rattle? This one can be used by an older child for whom 'baby' rattles are too small and fragile.

Rosemary uses a tough plastic salad shaker that looks like two colanders joined together by a hinge. Normally, freshly washed lettuce is placed inside and rapidly shaken to remove all the surplus water. Replace the lettuce with ping-pong balls or, better still, cat balls (each with a bell inside) from the pet shop. Tie the two halves of the salad shaker together. Bind round the handles and tie at intervals round the edge. You now have a large, strong rattle that can be carried about or hung up to be biffed or kicked.

A Slither Box

Quick

This rattle makes an unusual sound. It is used in the sound picture described on p. 57 to imitate the noise of footsteps on gravel. Tilted more slowly, it can make you think of waves breaking on a stony beach. It contains fish grit (used in aquaria), and the feeling of the weight being transferred from one hand to the other is intriguing to children. When one boy first held it, he spent ages slowly turning it over and over in an attempt to make a continuous sound. Its unusual shape and sound makes it attractive to older children who have thoroughly explored the possibilities of other percussion instruments. Be generous with the papier mâché layers that cover it and it will be very strong.

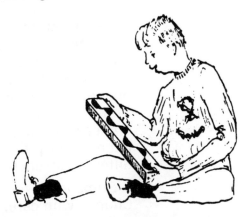

Use a fairly large *flat* cardboard box—the longer the better. Put in a few spoonfuls of fish grit or, for the softer sound, use rice, dried peas, etc.—experiment! Next, thoroughly cover the box with many layers of strips of torn newspaper and PVA adhesive, watered down for economy! Wait for the box to be thoroughly dry. Cover the newsprint with a coat of pale emulsion paint. When that is dry, decorate the box with a bold pattern using Humbrol enamel, or water-based paint, and add a final protective cover of polyurethane varnish.

TOYS WITH AN INBUILT NOISE

Scrunch Bags

Instant or quick

As the name implies, these are simply bags (of any size) filled with something that will make a sound when they are squeezed.

For an instant one …

- Buy a net full of walnuts. Eat a few so that the remainder will have room to rattle around inside the net. Close the net securely.

- Use a small cushion cover with a zip fastener opening. Stuff it loosely with plastic packaging, such as the little trays used to separate jam tarts. Make sure the zip cannot come undone. (A few strategically placed stitches?)
- Find an odd sock—without holes, and long if possible. Put something scrunchy in the foot. Tie a knot in the top of the leg.

For a set of scrunch bags that look more like a proper toy, make several covers from strong material—not too thick or the sound of scrunching will be muffled. I sometimes use ripstop nylon offcuts from a kite manufacturer, or lycra trimmings from a maker of sports wear, but cotton or unbleached calico will do just as well. For added interest, vary the shapes of the bags and insert a different 'scrunch' in each. Close up the bag securely.

Some ideas for fillings:
Choose with care. If the worst happens and the bag splits, contents which may be perfectly safe for the child in question might be dangerous for his friend (or the puppy!)

- A squeaky toy
- Round nuts that will slide about inside the bag
- A few *large* buttons
- Plastic packaging—crisp bags, sweet wrappers, cereal packet bags, bubble wrap, etc.
- Dry butter beans, peas, etc. for small bags—*not* lima beans or any other exotic seeds that need boiling to make them non-poisonous.
- Survival blanket—from an outdoor pursuits or camping shop.

A Chain in a Bottle

Almost instant

Hettie Whitby,
Teacher of Visually
Impaired Children

This is a simple but intriguing toy—one of the best I have come across. If you are familiar with Winnie-the-Pooh and his friends, you will know the story of Eeyore's birthday present. Pooh and Piglet meant to give him a jar of honey and a balloon, but one got accidentally popped and the other absentmindedly eaten. He ended up with a damp bit of rubbery rag and an empty honey jar. To his infinite satisfaction

Eeyore found that he could put the popped balloon in the honey jar, *and* take it out again! His friends left him happily repeating this action over and over again. This toy has the same appeal—now you see it, now you don't!

The bottle is a discarded plastic one that has a handle moulded into it. In its working life, it probably contained fabric softener. It is a pretty blue and, of course, the handle makes it easy to grasp. The chain can be bought from the local ironmongers (or DIY store). The length needed is about twice the height of the bottle. In theory, the chain should stick to the bottom of the bottle with a blob of Araldite. I must confess mine did not. Perhaps the bottle was damp! It was a simple matter to stitch the chain to the bottom of the bottle by squinting through the neck and poking a long needle, threaded with button thread, in through one side of the bottle, through the end link and out of the other side. I repeated the process several times, in effect binding the chain to the bottom of the bottle. A child can have fun dropping the chain in the bottle and shaking it out again but, for most children, it is better to go one step further and tie a ring or a cotton reel to the other end of the chain. This makes is easy to hold and prevents it from totally disappearing inside the bottle. Offer this peculiar toy to a child who has just learnt to sit independently, or to an older one who has a craze on 'doodle' toys, and you are sure to have a happy and satisfied customer!

Octopully

Long-lasting

A short entry in an early edition of Information Exchange described how an enterprising teacher in a Special Care Unit filled old tights with crunched-up newspaper and draped them over the children. What a splendid 'instant' idea—surely it could be developed into an attractive long-lasting toy!

The multi-armed octopus seemed the ideal model for such a toy, and soon the usual hotch potch of materials was transformed into the Octopully. Unlike the real thing, this version has tentacles that are

63

intended to be explored by inquisitive fingers and, on the end of each, is a bag containing a rattle, squeaker, bell, etc. It has been given the 'thumbs up' by children with multiple disabilities, who have obligingly tested it for me.

The Octopully can be hung up (possibly on elastic to make it more challenging to grab), tied to the side of a cot, draped across a play table, or just left lying about on the floor to be discovered by a child who, in all probability, will feel motivated to roll, 'swim' or crawl towards it.

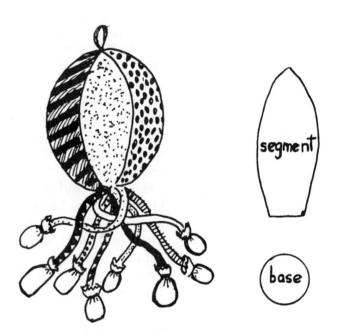

Materials
- Scraps of material for the body and for the bags at the end of the tentacles.
- Short length of piping or nylon cord for the hanging loop.
- Polyester filling.
- Small circle of card for the base of the body.
- Lengths of material for the tentacles could be:
  wide, strong ribbon, flat or plaited;
  thick wool, plaited;

bubbly plastic, cut in strips about 5cm (2")
wide and plaited;

a string of large beads loosely threaded on
nylon cord;

pyjama cord or wool braid, decorated with
buttons firmly sewn on;

stitched tubes of material with a pleasant feel
and/or bright colour. (Seam together the long
edges of a strip of material, right side inside.
Attach a safety pin to one end, poke it in the
tube and gradually work it along until it
comes out at the other end, turning the tube
the right side out in the process);

anything else you can think of!

● A selection of noisemakers in containers for the
tentacle ends, see list of suggestions p. 68.

Method

Refer to the diagram and make a paper pattern. A
suitable size for the body of the Octopully is about
20cm (8") long. Using strong, brightly-coloured
material, cut out six body segments. Stitch them
together, stopping just short of the top. By doing
this, you will have left a small hole for the insertion
of the hanging loop. Push the ends of the loop into
the hole and knot them together inside the body. By
hand, neaten the top of the Octopully. Turn in any
raw edges and sew round it several times. This will
also make sure that the loop will never pull out.

Make eight tentacles (suggested size 30cm or 12")
and sew them to the open end of the Octopully.

Cut out the circular base in card, and cover it with a
larger circle of material. Keep the material in position
with a few criss-crossing threads (which will be
hidden inside the body once the base is attached).

Now stuff the Octopully with polyester fibre, then
close the hole with the circular base, keeping it in
place with at least two rounds of ladder stitch.

Make eight bags for the ends of the tentacles. Fill
them with noisemakers of your choice and stitch one
(firmly!) to the end of each tentacle.

A Friendly Rattlesnake

Long-lasting

A few years ago I was asked to make some toys for some overseas children I had never met. I knew they had learning difficulties and were all under five; also that there might be times during the day when the play would be unsupervised. Therefore, a toy that was as strong and as safe as possible was required. After various experiments, I came up with an impressively long snake that was both noisy and tactile.

At the time my 'grot box' contained some tough plastic pill bottles with safety caps. Putting a few dried peas in one of these gave it an instant rattle with a splendid clatter. The skin of the snake was made from pieces of strong material joined together patchwork fashion. I began to experiment, and found that a snake which had eaten an exclusive diet of pill bottles was too noisy. Of course, this could be a good point for a child with a hearing loss, but I was considering the nerves of the adults! This is why the 'feely' sections were introduced. I soon had a production line going, and a box full of friendly snakes. Someone visiting the children reported that, after about three months' heavy use, they were grubby, but still intact.

Materials
- Small pieces of very strong, colourful fabric for the skin.
- A little polyester fibre for the head and the tail.
- A collection of tactile objects. Select suitable ones from the list on p. 89.
- Some rattles, and other noisemakers. Suggestions for fillings on p. 68.

Method

Make the snake about a metre long. This gives plenty of scope for interesting 'innards'. Lay out the contents of the snake in the order in which you will use them, grading them in size. Alternate a tactile section with a noisy one. Arrange the different pieces of fabric in an attractive way, possibly putting a narrow strip of the same colour between each. I found this gave the snake a pleasing appearance and acted as a hinge between the sections, making the toy suitably floppy. When the time came to fill the snake, I left these strips empty.

Next, cut each section of fabric the right size to fit the article it will later contain—large things near the head, graduating down towards the tail. Each section of fabric must be wide enough to wrap round a hard, unyielding rattle, with a bit extra for the seam allowance. The length of each piece will vary.

Rattles should fit fairly snugly inside their section, but tactile objects should have room to move around, as in a feely bag. Don't forget the seam allowance at each end, where one section joins the next. Join all the pieces of fabric together in a long strip. Fold this in half, right sides together, and pin at all the places where the fabrics join. Round off the head and the tail of the snake. Stitch along the side seam and round the end of the tail. Turn the snake skin right side out. Stuff the tail with polyester fibre. Stitch across the snake skin to keep it in place. (If you have used narrow strips of unifying fabric between the sections, as in the illustration, stitch across again just before the next section.) Continue like this, adding the contents as you go. Finally, stuff the head with polyester fibre, close the seam with ladder stitch and add felt features to give the snake a benign expression.

Noisy Busy Board

Long-lasting

This is a toy with plenty of scope for ingenuity. Basically, it is just a sheet of sturdy ply, whatever shape and size you choose, with an assortment of noisemakers screwed to it. Some, like the motor horn and the bicycle bell in the illustration, might

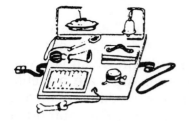

need a firm touch to set them going; others, like the bell and the bone scraper, can give a noisy reward for less physical effort. The number of items on the board, their spacing, simplicity and noisiness can all be governed by the needs of the child in question. A wander round the pet shop, DIY store or local iron-mongers is sure to produce plenty of attractive noisemakers suitable for mounting. For anyone with an electrical bent, a battery-driven bell or a morse buzzer could be included.

See also
   Fiddle Toys, p. 85.
   Amorphous Beanbag, p. 88.
   A Manx Feely Cushion, p. 89.

LIST OF NOISEMAKERS

This list is suitable for use in homemade rattles or noisy toys. *Consider the safety factor* and select carefully for the child in mind.

- Beads
- Bells, various sizes and shapes. From craft shops, pet shops, etc.
- Buttons, the larger the better for safety reasons
- Butterbeans
- Dried peas
- Film cartons. Suitable contents inserted and lid taped on before sewing inside a toy
- Fish grit, from pet shops
- Foil milk bottle tops
- Pill bottles with safety caps. Suitable contents inside
- Potato crisp packets for scrunchy paper
- Rice
- Sound buttons. Squeeze one and it plays a tune. From craft suppliers
- Squeakers, from craft shops, etc.
- Squeaky toys, use the whole toy inside, e.g. the Friendly Rattlesnake or Octopully.

LISTENING GAMES

Echoes

Instant

This can be a good game to play at odd moments, on car journeys, etc. It consists of imitating a familiar sound like a clock ticking, a fire engine, a car hooter or an animal noise. You make the sound and your child echoes it. Then, perhaps, he makes the sound for you to copy. Making a noise to produce a real echo, (in a valley, or walking through a tunnel?) can prompt a child to listen really intently.

Rattles in Pairs to make a Sound Matching Game

Quick

Collect an even number of containers with lids—at least six. Film cartons, little plastic pots (used to hold potato salad, etc.) or even a collection of Nesquick tins, might do. Whatever you use, it is essential that the containers are identical, and that the contents will be invisible. Arrange the containers in pairs, and put a small quantity of the same noisemaker in each pair. Replace the lids and glue or tape them on. The containers are muddled up, and placed in line on the table. The children take it in turns to choose two, shake them, and hope that they will match in sound. If they do not, the containers are returned to the same places on the table, and someone else tries his luck. An observant child who has been listening hard will notice which sound each container has made and, when his turn comes, will probably be able to pick a pair.

Suitable fillings for the containers might be rice, dried peas, butter beans, pebbles, coins, bells, buttons, sand, or milk bottle tops. It is important that the pairs of sounds are distinguishable from each other. Rice and lentils, shaken in the same kind of container can sound identical. Consider the safety factor very carefully when using items from this list. You know best the habits of the children who will use your game, and if they are likely to remove the lids and make a meal of the contents.

This sound matching game can be interesting for any age from toddler to teenager. At the younger end, make the sounds very distinctive and not too numerous. Use, for example, sand, bells and dried peas. At the older end, use more pairs of sounds and make them less easily distinguishable. Some teenagers are likely to be curious about the contents of the containers, and with their stronger hands may easily remove the lids. This was certainly the case with one group. No known glue could defeat them! The problem was solved by covering the containers, in this case film cartons, with strips of newspaper and paste. When dry, they were all painted the same colour. The children could no longer *see* the lids, so the urge to take them off disappeared.

Note
I have recently made a 'starter kit' for this game. It is for young children, or perhaps slightly older ones with learning difficulties. As in the game above, identical containers have been used. Film cartons again! These are strong, just the right size for small hands— and free! (My local chemist soon collects me a carrier bag full.) I make use of only two sounds and divide them equally among, say, twelve film cartons. The child's task is to rattle them, one by one, listen to the sound and separate them into sets of six. This game is a winner if preceded by a little story. Supposing the noisemakers used are rice and fish grit. The story might be about some pirates who hid their treasure in a cave. In order to confuse anyone coming across it they put sand (rice) in some of the containers and gold coins (fish grit!) in the others. Find the treasure and sort it out!

Of course, the lids must be firmly fixed on the film cartons. Adhesives will not do the job properly. Adhesive tape can be safe in certain circumstances, but I tape the lids in position and *then* put the whole carton safely inside a serviceable dark blue crochet cover (as with the Roller Rattle p. 60).

Musical Bumps

This is a good group game for letting off steam. While the music plays, the children jiggle about on the spot. When the music stops, they must sit on the floor. (All that getting up and down can be quite exhausting!) When played as a party game, the last child to sit down is 'out', and the best listener who always drops to the floor first is rewarded with a small prize. If the group is small, I prefer to play the game non-competitively, and give everyone their share of praise.

Musical Statues

This is yet another version of the musical start-stop game. The children dance around and, when the music stops, they must instantly become a statue, and keep absolutely still until the music starts again. This calls for considerable balancing skill. You can either withdraw the first child that wobbles, or play uncompetitively and praise the best statue. To praise is kinder and usually leads to more imaginative efforts and greater fun.

BODY AWARENESS AND TICKLING GAMES

Children who are lying down are in a perfect position to benefit from this kind of play. Take 'Body Awareness' first. Children with a visual impairment may not be able to see the various parts of their bodies, so it is possible they may not even be aware that they are there. Daily care routines provide the ideal opportunities to focus on feet, hands, knees, elbows, etc. Drying in between toes to the accompaniment of 'This little piggy went to market' can be part of the bathtime ritual—after many repetitions, the child learns to anticipate the punch line when the last little piggy 'Goes wee, wee, wee, all the way home'. Often the best body awareness games are those made up on the spur of the moment to fit a particular situation. For instance, take nappy-changing time. This is the moment when babies revel in the feeling of freedom and will take the opportunity to have a good old kick. One mother invented this simple formula. She cradled her son's heels in the palms of her hands, helping him to make leisurely cycling movements as she said, 'Slowly - slowly - up the hill' ... after a pause for dramatic effect came the climax when together they 'cycled' rapidly to the words, 'And down the other side'. This ritual could be repeated ten times and still he would want it again!

71

Spontaneous tickling games are one of the joys of babyhood. They work best when adult and child are relaxed and enjoying each other's company. The adult gives the child a gentle tickle, perhaps on her cheek, and is rewarded with smiles and chuckles.

Now for some body-awareness and tickling rhymes which may jog your memory, or increase your repertoire.

This little piggy went to market, *(waggle big toe)*.
This little piggy stayed at home, *(waggle the next toe)*.
This little piggy ate roast beef.
This little piggy had none, *(pause for effect)*.
This little piggy cried 'wee, wee, wee' all the way home, *(by now you should have reached the last and smallest toe)*.

Round and round the garden, like a teddy bear, *(describe small circles on the palm of the child's hand,)*
One step, two step, *(walk your fingers up his arm to the rhythm cf the words),*
And tickle me under there! *(Tickle under chin, under arm, etc.)*

Two little eyes to look around,
Two little ears to hear each sound,
One little nose to smell what's sweet,
One little mouth that likes to eat.
(Touch each feature gently as it is mentioned.)

Shoe the little horse,
Shoe the little mare,
But let the little colt
Go bare, bare, bare,
(Pat soles of baby's feet in rhythm to the words.)

Heads and shoulders, knees and toes, knees and
toes, knees and toes,
Heads and shoulders knees and toes, we all clap
hands together.

Tickle bird, Tickle bird, fly to *(child's name)* ears
*(Run fingers up the child's body and gently tickle his
ears.)*
*Repeat for other parts of the child's body. Pause
between tickles for dramatic effect! End up with ...*
Tickle here, tickle there, tickle EVERYWHERE!

Slowly, slowly, very slowly, creeps the garden snail,
Slowly, slowly, very slowly, up the garden rail.
Quickly, quickly, very quickly, runs the little mouse,
Quickly, quickly, very quickly, round about the house.
(Make your tickling fingers suit the words.)

Rocking Rhymes

See-saw, Marjory Dawe, Jenny shall have a new
master.
She shall earn but a penny a day because she can't
work any faster.
*(Sit the child on your knee, or between your legs on
the floor. Hold hands and rock gently together, back-
wards and forwards, in time to the words.)*

Row, row, row the boat, gently down the stream,
Merrily, merrily, merrily, merrily, life is just a dream!
*(Sit on the floor, facing each other. Hold hands and
rock to and fro, in unison as above.)*

Bye, Baby Bunting, Daddy's gone a-hunting
Gone to find a rabbit skin to wrap the Baby Bunting
in.
(Rock child in your arms in time to the words.)

Hush-a-bye baby, on the tree top.
when the wind blows the cradle will rock.
When the bough breaks the cradle will fall,
And down will come baby, cradle and all.
(Another traditional rhyme for rocking a child in your arms.)

Jingles for a Child Sitting on Your Knee

(Sit the child facing you and hold his hands.)
This is the way the farmer rides,
plod, plod, plod;
(Roll the child slowly from side to side as though riding a cart horse)
This is the way the lady rides,
Trit trot, trit trot, trit trot;
(Jiggle the child up and down to the trotting rhythm)
This is the way the gentleman rides,
Gallopy, gallopy, gallopy;
(Make your knee movements as high as you dare!)
And FALLS into a ditch.
(On FALLS hold the child extra firmly and let him slide between your legs.)

To market, to market to buy a fat pig,
Home again, home again,
Jiggerty jig.

To market, to market to buy a fat hog,
Home again, home again,
Joggerty jog.
(Slow jogs from side to side for the first two lines. Quick jogs for the last lines.)

Leg over, leg over, the dog went to Dover.
When he came to a style, JUMP, he went over.
(Rock slowly from side to side to side. Lift up on jump.)

74

Bell horses, bell horses, what time of day?
One o'clock, two o'clock, three and AWAY.
*(Hold child's hands securely and jiggle him up and
down in time to the rhythm of the words. On AWAY let
him slip between your knees.)*

Father and Mother and Uncle John
Went to market, one by one.
Father fell off *(slip child to one side)*
And Mother fell off *(slip child to the other side)*
But Uncle John went on, and on, and on, and on ...

Jelly on the plate, jelly on the plate,
Wibble wobble, wibble wobble, jelly on the plate.

Learning to feel

FOR VISUALLY HANDICAPPED CHILDREN the senses of hearing and touch must obviously be developed as fully as possible to compensate for their impaired sight. The more the use of these senses can be encouraged, the quicker the child can become less dependent and lead a fuller life. The three-year-old with nimble fingers can sort her socks into pairs by feeling the patterns on the legs, and even tights can be put on with less of a battle if she can first sort out the gusset from the heels. Recognising toys by their feel, and realising where she is by touching the textured wallpaper or cold kitchen tiles are skills she will soon learn. As she grows older, she will gradually discover how to dress and undress herself, managing buttons, zips and poppers on the way. She will go shopping and learn to sort and identify coins, and at school she will learn Braille. For this she will need not only a good memory, but also very sensitive fingertips to help her distinguish between the various combinations of the six tiny dots which make up the Braille symbols. Such sensitivity may be helped by using the toys, activities and games that follow.

FOCUSING ON HANDS

Hands! What incredible appendages they are! Like our miraculous eyes and ears, we take them for granted. Consider the average day. Between getting up and going to bed, our hands will have helped us with washing, dressing, eating, turning knobs, holding things, writing—pen in hand or with modern technology—reading Braille ... this list of uses could fill this page. Hands are also a vital part of our body language. Through them we can reinforce the meaning of our words. Even one finger can be used to point to something for a child to fetch us, or it can be used in an admonishing manner—'Don't you *dare* do that again!' Our fingers might be compared to tentacles or feelers. We use them to grasp, pull, poke, twist, pick up tiny things and to hold and manipulate tools. No wonder we spend so much time helping the children in our care to make the best use of their hands.

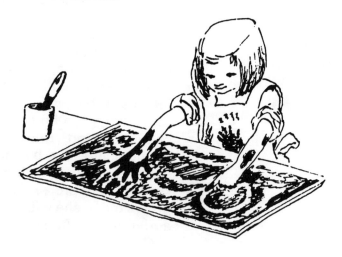

Hand Prints

Quick

People who work and play with brain-damaged children are often looking for new ways of encouraging them to focus on different parts of their bodies, and so help them to understand which bit does what! Making a hand (or foot) print is one way of concentrating a child's attention on that part of him. Hands can be smeared with a fairly thick mixture of powder paint and then used to print their shape on a piece of paper. Alternatively, each hand can be placed flat on the paper while you draw round it. The child can take his time, flattening out his hand and spreading his fingers. Then comes the best bit when he experiences a delightful tingling sensation as your pencil traces round his fingers. Try it!

Hand prints are often cut out and used for classroom decoration. At Linden Bennet School each child in the class makes several pairs of hand prints and a pair of foot prints. These are cut out and arranged on large sheets of paper as giant flowers. The foot prints, together with a photograph of the child go in the centre of the flower and the hand prints are arranged all around to make the petals.

At Dysart School the body of a large bird is drawn on sugar paper and the outline filled in with overlapping hand-prints, pointing towards the tail, to represent feathers.

At other schools cut-out hand prints are used to make very effective trees. In Autumn, they are made in red, yellow and brown to represent the seasonal colours. The hand prints are mounted on paper in the shape of a tree with the fingers pointing upwards. In December, there is a call for more hand prints, dark green this time. They can be mounted, fingers pointing downwards, to represent a Christmas tree.

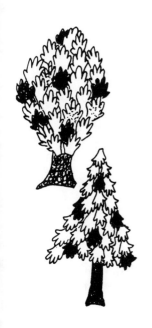

Zebra Play Mittens

The magical moment when a tiny baby discovers her fingers can make the day a red letter one. She has found these wonderful appendages which can bend, stretch and wiggle about. Soon she will learn to hold things for a closer inspection and guide them to her mouth for further exploration. Children with a visual

79

impairment sometimes miss out on this early hand play, because they are not aware their hands are there. A simple way of focusing attention on hands is to play tickling and clapping games (like 'Round and round the garden' *see* p. 72 and Pat-a-cake *see* p. 82) but there is a limit to the amount of time that can be spent this way. In an attempt to make a child's hands more noticeable, I have devised some simple mittens that cover the backs and palms of hands but leave the fingers and thumbs free. They have been very successful with children with partial sight and with some who also have hemiplegia and/or learning difficulties.

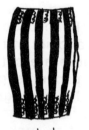

Style 1

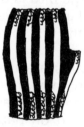

Style 2

Materials
- Small amounts of 4ply wool in contrasting colours. I use black and white and the directions are given accordingly.
- Knitting needles, size 3¼ (10).
- Wool needle.

Method
The pattern given will fit an average child of about 2–3 years old. For a larger child just add a few more stitches and rows!

Cast on 24 st. in black.
Row 1. K.
Row 2. K3 (for a non-curl 'collar' round the fingers) P14, K7 (for the cuff).
Row 3. Join in white and knit.
Row 4. As for row 2.
Rows 5 and 6. Repeat the first two rows.
Continue to make alternate black and white stripes until you have finished the fourth white stripe. (One for each finger.)
The thumb—Style one, making a slit.
Row 1. K black.
Row 2. K3, P14, K7.
Row 3. White. K12, cast off 6, K to end.
Row 4. K3, P3, cast on 6, P5, K7.
The thumb—Style two, making a gusset.
Row 1. K black.

Row 2. K3, P14, K7.
Row 3. K17, turn.
Row 4. K3, P3, turn.
Row 5. K6, turn.
Row 6. K3, P7, K7.
Row 7. White. K17, turn.
Row 8. K3, P7, K7.
Row 9. Black. K17, turn.
Row 10. K3, P3, turn.
Row 11. K6, turn.
Row 12. K3, P7, K7.
Row 13. K24.
Row 14. As row 2.

Repeat the black and white stripe pattern to match the half already made, remembering to keep the 'collar' and cuff borders even. End with a black stripe. Cast off and sew up the side seam.

Finger Plays and Clapping Rhymes

Roly poly ever so slowly, (rotate hands around each other)
Higher and higher,
Lower and lower,
Wider and wider,
Slower and slower,
And faster, and faster, and faster …

Here is the tree with leaves so green, (arms up, fingers spread)
Here are the apples that hang between, (make fists)
When the wind blows, the apples will fall.
Here is the basket to gather them all (link fingers).

Ten little men standing up straight, (palms together)
Ten little men open the gate, (open out hands, like reading a book)
Ten little men all in a ring, (cup hands together, fingers straight)
Ten little men bow to the king (bend fingers)
Ten little men dance all day, (wiggle fingers)
Ten little men hide away (put hands behind back).

Two fat gentlemen *(thumbs)* met in the lane,
Bowed most politely, bowed once again
Two thin ladies *(first fingers)* ...
Two tall policemen *(middle fingers)* ...
Two small schoolboys *(ring fingers)* ...
Two tiny babies *(little fingers)* ...

Five fat peas in a pea pod pressed, *(make a fist)*
One grew (poke out thumb), two grew *(poke out a finger)*
And so did all the rest *(open hand).*
They grew and they grew and they didn't stop *(stretch hands apart)*
'Till all of a sudden the pod went POP! *(Clap)*

Tommy Thumb, Tommy Thumb, where are you? *(hands behind back)*
Here I am (bring out one,) here I am *(bring out the other)*
How do you do? *(thumbs bow to each other)*

Repeat with
   Peter Pointer ...
   Middle Man ...
   Ruby Ring ...
   Baby Small ...
   Fingers all ...

Open them, shut them, open them, shut them,
Give a little clap,
Shut them, open them, shut them, open them,
Lay them in your lap.

Pat-a-cake, pat-a-cake, baker's man,
Bake me a cake as fast as you can.
Pat it and prick it and mark it with B
And put it in the oven for Baby and me.

Wind the bobbin up, wind the bobbin up,
Pull, pull, clap, clap, clap
Wind the bobbin up, wind the bobbin up,
Pull, pull, clap, clap, clap.
Point to the ceiling, point to the floor,
Point to the window, point to the door.
Put your hands together, one, two, three *(clap)*
Put your hands upon your knee.

Roly Poly, Roly Poly, up, up, up.
Roly Poly, Roly Poly, down, down, down.
Roly Poly, Roly Poly, clap, clap, clap,
Roly Poly, Roly Poly. Hands behind your back.

USING HANDS

Toys are all very well, but by far the best way of encouraging a child to use his hands is to involve him in daily life. What child can resist the delight of rolling out the pastry or squeezing the off-cuts into the shape of a pig? Don't succumb to temptation and put the grubby dolls clothes in the washing machine. Show your child how to wash them by hand— soaping, rinsing and squeezing (or wringing out) before pegging on a low-hung washing line. All time-consuming for the adult, but minutes well spent when you consider all that 'therapy' added to the fun and satisfaction the child has experienced.

Unwrapping the Contents of the Shopping Basket

This can be a very useful and informative occupation. Perhaps the shopping can be divided between two bags, one for fragile items and the other for packets and tins, which are safe for a toddler to handle. Through picking up the various items, he will learn a lot about size, weight, shape and possibly smell. He will have the fun of taking things out of bags, and can learn to recognise the contents by looking at the packaging. He may even be able to pick out special letters like his own initial. During all this inspection, his hands will have been turning the articles around, helping him to gain confidence in handling, but not dropping, them.

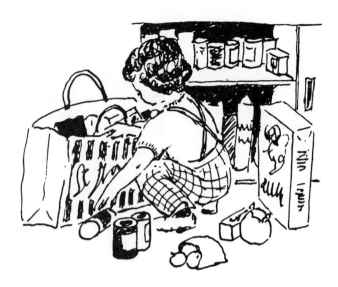

Hiding Things in Containers

An old handbag can make a perfect toy! Just fill it with a glorious conglomeration of feely articles; (large buttons; shiny, round conkers; an empty crisp packet; a squeaky toy; an odd sock with a bell tied in it—to name but a few.)

Some children like to wiggle their fingers in a bowl of sand, sawdust, rice, etc, to find a small hidden toy. Others like to fish in a bowl of soapsuds to find a surprise. This can be a good activity for bathtime. Put some bubblebath in a small basin. All the inevitable drips and splashes then fall harmlessly into the big bath where they can be put to their proper use!

Fiddle Toys

At every age it seems there are times when we love to 'fiddle'—handling something for the sheer pleasure we receive through our fingertips. Imagine sitting on a sunny beach sifting the dry sand through your fingers, or fiddling with an elastic band. I suppose even stroking the cat might sometimes be considered a 'fiddle'! Activities like these are relaxing and a pleasant tactile experience. Children are inveterate fiddlers, and usually find their own favourite objects. Some children with very special needs may not be able to choose for themselves and might appreciate a ready-made fiddle toy. Here are some suggestions.

A Serendipity of Fiddle Toys

Almost Instant - just allow a little time to collect them all!

Dr Lili Nielson, Danish expert on the education of visually impaired children

Lili Nielson has a magic suitcase full of bits and pieces, guaranteed to please any child with a passion for fiddling. With such motivation and busy fingers, plenty of tactile experiences are sure to follow! Lift the lid of the case and you will find ...

- about four strings of beads and buttons, joined together at one end so that the loose ends form a tassel;
- old bed springs, with the ends bent in and protected with sticky tape;
- a pliable soap saver with little plastic suckers on the reverse side;
- a bunch of real keys on a strong ring, with a wooden tag to dangle them by;
- an embroidery frame with tracing paper stretched tightly over it, making it like a flat little drum;
- an electric toothbrush holder, battery driven and without the brush, to switch on and off, so experiencing the pleasant vibration;
- three long strands of material, loosely plaited together, so that small fingers can wiggle between the strands;
- a bunch of Bendy Straws, taped together at the long ends, so that the bendy parts at the other end can be twisted about in different directions;
- large buttons on a loop of elastic;
- plenty of rattles and tins to shake.

One can imagine any child saying to itself; 'Just let me get at that lot!'

Tactile Bags

Quick

These are made like beanbags, but the contents are chosen for their variety and tactile appeal. Ideally, the covers should be fairly thin, so that the contents are easily felt through the fabric, but can't be seen. The idea is to put at least two articles in each bag, so that the child can separate them out by wiggling them about inside. As usual, select items suitable for the group or child in mind. For children with sharp teeth, it may be necessary to use tougher material. Stitch round the seams several times and be extra fussy about closing the gap once the contents are inside. If, in spite of all your efforts, there is any chance that the bags might possibly be opened, make sure the contents will do no harm if eaten. Here are some possible fillings to start you off.

- A slightly inflated balloon and a ping-pong ball.
- Rice and a few large buttons.
- Two curtain rings and some dried peas.
- Orange pips and a marble.
- A cotton reel, some coins or sponge rubber.

Grab Bags

Instant or Quick

These are just an enlarged and tougher version of the tactile bags above. They are intended to be used by children with an iron grip, and are useful for hanging on many of the toy supports suggested in the section on Keeping Toys Within Reach (p. 9).

For an instant version, use the strong net bags used to package oranges, onions, etc. Partly fill the net with conkers or acorns, in season, or nuts, or shiny, crunchy plastic packaging from a box of tarts—and there you are!

For the quick version, you might start off with a small tin. Inside put bells from a broken toy, buttons, or a few grains of rice, etc. Glue or tape on the lid and enclose the tin in a bag made from brightly coloured, very strong fabric. (Upholstery material, deck chair canvas, kite material ... *see* list on p. 91.)

Tactile Tortoise

Long-lasting

This strange animal was first made for a small girl with Cerebral Palsy, and before long it became her favourite toy.

I have made several since the prototype and all have enticed idle fingers to be busy. One particular success story was with a teenager in the hospital school where I then worked. She had severe learning difficulties, poor sight and limited movement in her hands. It was difficult to persuade her to join in any of the activities on offer. She only came to life at meal times! One day, in desperation, I put a tactile tortoise on her knee. It was quite heavy—having been well filled with chopped-up tights (for economy!). For this girl the weight was important for she could not ignore the strange object now resting on her knees. During the sing-song that concluded the afternoon, we noticed that her fingers were beginning to explore all the little cushions on the back of the tortoise. Once she found the tail filled with marbles, that was it!

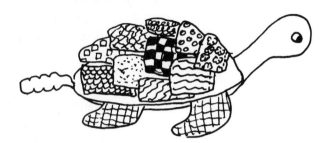

Materials

- Strong material for the body, e.g. tweed, upholstery material.
- Thin material in different colours for the little bags that cover the tortoise's back, and also form the legs and tail.
- Tactile objects to put inside the bags. *See* list on p. 89 for suggestions.
- Scraps of felt for features.
- Stuffing for the head and body. Polyester filling or chopped-up tights.

Method

In the strong material, cut out the underside of the body. Make it oval and about 30cm (12") long. Cut out a second oval, slightly larger. This will be humped up to make the curved back of the tortoise.

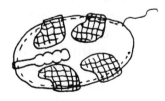

Make several small bags in the thinner material (say eight or ten) and put various tactile objects inside. Arrange the bags on the larger oval (leaving a generous seam allowance round the edge) and machine stitch them in place. (They are supposed to represent the sections of the tortoise's shell!) Make four more bags for the floppy legs and feet (sock shape) and put something tactile in each of them. Tack across the top to prevent the contents from spilling out when you assemble the tortoise. To represent the tail, make a fabric tube. Stretch material is best. Stitch across one end, and put in about four marbles. Leave space between them, so that they can be moved about within the tail. Tack across the open end.

Make a neck and head as in the illustration and stuff it firmly. Put this part aside while the rest of the tortoise is assembled. On the *right* side of the under-body pin the legs in position, *facing inwards*. Pin the tail at the back, but make it point towards where the head will be. Gather round the top section of the tortoise, so that it will fit the underbody. Leaving a gap for turning (where the head will go) pin and tack the shell to the underside, making sure the feely parts (shell segments, legs and tail) are tucked inside. Sew the top to the bottom. Turn the whole thing inside out and you should have a deflated, headless tortoise! Stuff the body firmly, then push the neck into the opening and sew it securely in place with several rounds of ladder stitching. The head makes a convenient handle and will take a lot of strain. If it tends to flop forward, adjust the stitching until it is as you want it.

Bear in mind the tortoise is not easily washed, especially if you have used pasta or rice in the feely bags! It is best kept as a special treasure for an individual child.

Amorphous Beanbag

Quick

Sylvia O'Bryan,
Tutor,
Toymaking

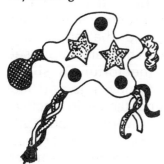

As its name suggests, this beanbag is a wholly unconventional shape. This, of course, is part of its attraction. The body of the beanbag is about the size of a tea plate, but its shape is anything but circular. At two places the material is extended into pairs of 'prongs' which narrow towards their ends and finish with dangling plaits of textured material or bunches of ribbon—lovely to slide between the fingers. The top of the bag is cut slightly larger than the bottom, and a small pocket is inserted roughly in the middle, like the crater of a volcano! This is lined with fur fabric and gathered up with elastic so that an exploring finger can poke around inside. The beanbag is lightly stuffed with dried peas which can be manoeuvred in and out of the 'prongs'. Sylvia obviously has considerable needlework skills, but an

Amorphous Beanbag, without the pocket, is no more difficult to make than the conventional and uninteresting (one might even say boring) square or oblong shape. Think of a treasure island with lots of bays and peninsulas and make a beanbag like that. The children will love it!

A Manx Feely Cushion

Quick

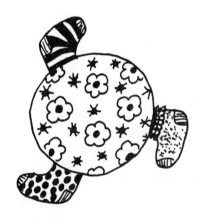

This circular cushion, like the emblem for the Isle of Man, has three legs. In this case they are made from small, brightly-coloured socks, each with a tactile or noisemaking object inside, stitched at equal distances round the edge of the cushion. To make it, just cut out two circles of fabric with a pleasant feel, (velvet? fur fabric?) about the size of a dinner plate, and fill three small socks with something tactile or noisy, (*see* list below and on p. 68 for suggestions). Tack across the top of the socks to keep the contents inside. Put the circles of material right sides together and arrange the socks (pointing inwards) with their tops at equal intervals around the edges of the circles. Pin and tack them in place. Sew most of the way round the edge of the cushion (twice) leaving a gap for turning and stuffing. Turn the cushion right side out and stuff the centre with polyester fibre or crunchy paper—or what you will. Close the gap securely.

Suggestions for Contents of Tactile Bags

Safety First! Consider carefully the child or children you have in mind before selecting any of the materials on the following list. Something that may be perfectly justifiable and stimulating for one child may be unsuitable—and possibly even dangerous—for another. Some children will always find an inappropriate way of using a toy, and I am sure all readers can think of their own cautionary tales. Vigilance and common sense are the basic essentials for safety, so please use plenty of common sense when selecting from these suggestions. The choice is yours!

Beads–large
Bricks—wooden or plastic
Buttons—large
Cotton reels

Crunchy plastic, e.g. packaging tray from a box of
    jam tarts, or paper, e.g. crisp packet
Curtain rings—large
Fish grit
Lolly sticks
Nylon pan scrubber
Plastic shapes from a mosaic, etc
Polyester fibre for a soft feel
Rattle
Rice, etc. (won't wash!)
Real objects, e.g. spoon, comb, tooth-brush, etc.
Shells—large
Smartie tops
Squeaky toy

See also
Chain in a Bottle, p. 62

EXPLORING TEXTURES

Just Feeling

Very Quick

Sylvia O'Bryan suggests stitching a soft piece of material (e.g. fur fabric) *inside* a child's pocket. Every time he puts his hand in, he will experience the pleasant texture.

Alison Harland collects together several brightly-coloured pairs of tights, and ties them together to make an exotic octopus. Each leg is stuffed with a different 'feel'. This might be scrunched-up newspaper, plastic foam pipe insulating wrap, ping-pong balls, etc. This wonderful creature can be hung from the ceiling hook, but Alison finds it is more fun to drape it over a couple of children, so that they can play tug-of-war.

Angela Smith (teacher of children with severe learning difficulties) keeps, in her stock cupboard, an extra large bag crammed to the top with tactile objects, ready for the daily 'feely' session. She includes vinyl squeaky toys, soft toys, wooden objects, a small cushion cover filled with plastic packaging, a tin mug—for its cold feel. She saves plastic net bags from the greengrocer and half fills them with pecan nuts, or milk bottle tops, plastic ribbon from the florist, or anything else she thinks will interest the children. She also runs a neat line in the quickest and easiest feely bags it is possible to make! She collects odd socks, puts in a few acorns, or corks, or large buttons—whatever comes to hand— ties a knot in the top of the leg ... and that is all there is to it!

A Feely Trail Along the Wall

Long-lasting

Seen at a Unit for Young Deaf/Blind Children

This 100% tactile snake wound its way along a corridor wall linking the reception area to the play room. With its help the children could find their way independently from one to the other. It might be an idea worth copying in a domestic situation, where it could be both decorative and helpful in guiding a child from one place to another—even up the stairs—and it would save grubby finger-marks along the wall!

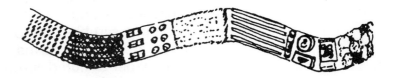

The snake in the unit was made from many pieces of card, (approximately 10 × 20cm—4 × 8") and covered with this imaginative collection of textures.

- Assorted pasta shapes
- Bunches of tissues sprinkled with perfume
- Buttons
- Carpeting
- Cornflakes
- Fur fabric
- Rice
- Sandpaper
- Scotchbrite scourer
- Shiny card
- Strips of macaroni
- Velvet
- Woolly balls

Materials With Tactile Appeal

The following list of suggestions may start you thinking:

Artificial grass—as seen at the greengrocers
Blanket, woolly ordinary weave, or the lanaircell type
　　with holes in

Bubbly plastic—large or small 'bubbles'. Used in packaging and can usually be had for the asking or can be bought at some large stationers and DIY stores

Carpet samples

Chain, metal or plastic, in many sizes. Ironmongers or DIY stores—or garden centres for the plastic kind

Coarse tweed

Corduroy

Felt

Fur fabric, long and short pile. (Make sure this won't pull out.)

Hessian

Needlecord

Nylon deck chair canvas

Nylon netting, many mesh sizes. Try curtaining shops or garden centres for a strong, large-meshed netting

Nylon pan scrubber, various shapes

Paper, in its many forms, from tissue to embossed wallpaper or fluted cardboard

Plastic foam from specialist shop or street market

PVC

Prickly doormat

Rug canvas from craft shop

Sandpaper, various grades

Satin

Survival blanket from sports shop, in the outdoor activities section

Taffeta

Terry towelling

Velvet

Vivelle (felt flocked paper from educational suppliers, p. 4)

TEXTURE MATCHING

Tactile Cubes

Long-lasting

These feely cubes were created for a small group of visually impaired children who also had learning difficulties. I was asked by their teacher to make them a toy with fairly large tactile surfaces. As it happened, I was looking for a way to recycle some clean, but shabby foam bricks. An obvious step seemed to be to recover the foam bricks, using a different texture for each face. They could be kept in a shallow box and used for matching and sorting. Pieces of fur fabric, PVC, velvet, 'bubbly' plastic (used in packaging), a rough tweed and corduroy were the textures selected. Then a square cardboard template was cut, very slightly smaller than the face of the cube. (If it was the same size the cover could turn out to be a sloppy fit, and the cube would end up a bad shape.) The template was used six times on each piece of textured fabric. The first square was drawn, then a gap left for seam allowances before the second square was marked out ... and so on, until all six squares were ready for cutting out. The marking lines were useful as seam lines when it came to joining all the squares together. I found the easiest way of doing this was to lay out all the six piles of different textures in a line. I took a square from each of the first two piles and stitched them together, leaving a small gap at the beginning and end of the seam. (This was necessary for making an accurate fit when the top and bottom squares were added.) I repeated the process until all the squares from the first two piles were paired together. Then, to each pair, I added a square from the third pile. To each strip of three I added the fourth texture. I pinned the ends together, forming a cube without its top or bottom. A square from the fifth pile was sewn to the top of the nearly finished cube, and the process repeated for all the other five. The final squares were stitched to all the bottoms. The pins were removed and the foam bricks forced into their new covers. A knitting needle was useful for persuading them into the corners. The last seams were closed by hand.

In play, the cubes could be turned over within the box until all the faces with the same texture were on top. Fur fabric was the easiest to identify, bubbly plastic the most popular! It did not matter if the children sorted by touch or sight. Once the cubes were correctly arranged, they could run their hands across the top and experience a large area of the same texture. Some learnt to make simple patterns with perhaps two textures arranged alternately as on a chess board, or in rows to make stripes.

Feely Caterpillar

Long-lasting

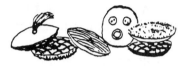

This peculiar creature consists of a series of little cushions joined together with Velcro circles. The back half of one cushion matches in texture the front half of the next, and so the fabrics correspond, domino fashion all along the caterpillar. The toy is popular with children—I suspect that is because of the ripping sound the Velcro makes!

Materials

- Fabrics with different textures, say six.
- A saucer to use as a template for cutting out the circles.
- A pack of Velcoins—Velcro circles, slightly larger than Velcro Spot-ons.
- A little polyester fibre for stuffing.
- Scraps of felt or buttons for the features.
- A small amount of wool for the tail. (Yes, *this* caterpillar has one!)

Method

Using the saucer as a template, draw two circles on the wrong side of each piece of material. Cut out the circles. Arrange them in pairs, in a row in front of you. Take a circle from the first pair and give it a face. (Perhaps button eyes and a curtain ring mouth.) Put it back at the head of the row. Take its twin and give it a tassel tail. Put it at the far end of the row. Take a circle from the next pair of textures and sew a Velcoin to the centre. Pin it to the back of the face—wrong sides together for the moment, so that you can see how the sequence of textures works out. Sew the other half of the Velcoin to the matching circle. Back it with a circle from the next pair (Velcoin attached). Continue in this way, matching texture to texture until you reach the tail. The sequence of textures should be perfect, (AB:BC:CD:D ... A). At this stage it is sensible to check that the Velcro coupling also works, and that you have not inadvertently put two of the same kind on one segment of the caterpillar.

Now to make up the caterpillar. Start with the head. Remove the pins, put the right sides together, tack and sew most of the way round, leaving a gap for turning and stuffing. Turn, lightly stuff and close the gap. Continue like this all down the line of cushions. Velcro them together as you go to check that all is well.

'Feely' Mitts

Quick

(Especially suitable for children with severe visual impairment)

Sorting mitt shapes into pairs can be a useful introduction to other tactile games. The shapes are large, so there is plenty of surface to feel. The pairing process is not as easy as you might think, especially for children who are not yet acquainted with a range of textile textures. If there are many pairs of mitts, the sorting out can be quite difficult. Sighted children (wearing blindfolds?) can also take part.

Collect some pieces of cardboard—old cereal packets will do—and a selection of textured fabrics. Place a child's hand on the cardboard and arrange it so that the fingers are together and the thumb slightly apart (mitt shape). Draw round it and cut it out. Repeat the process with the other hand. Use PVA adhesive and stick one pair of 'mitts' to the wrong side of each piece of textured material. Wait for the adhesive to dry, then cut off the surplus material.

During my teaching days I invented this activity for a bright little girl of five who had recently lost her sight. Once she could identify the pairs by touch, I expanded the game by putting eyelets in the cuffs of the mitts and showing her how to join the pairs together with treasury tags. This was a useful threading exercise, and probably helped her when it came to learning to insert shoelaces.

TACTILE BOOKS

Rustly Book

Quick

As a toy librarian I was used to searching among all the toys to find just the right one for a particular child, but one day I drew a blank. I needed a plaything for a little girl who had learning difficulties, a hearing loss, was partially sighted and also had difficulty in using her hands. Quite a challenge for a toy librarian! Every toy suggested had either been borrowed several times before, or was unsuitable in some way. Fortunately, her mother discovered a toy I had overlooked, so she did not leave the toy library empty handed. I promised to try to be creative before her next visit.

We needed a toy which combined noise, movement, colour and a pleasant feel. It should also be safe, strong, and washable. Difficult! It so happened the packer had been generous with the bubbly plastic protecting the last lot of toys received at the toy library, so that could make a starting point. Children love this material for its texture, the rustly noise it makes and the joy of popping the 'bubbles'.

I used this material to make a bag like a small cushion cover, and put a few large, brightly-coloured buttons inside. The result was attractive, but of limited appeal. It could be shaken about and the buttons would make a clicking sound as they moved inside the bag, but then what? Several more bags were run up on the sewing machine and different fillings were put in each. I now had a collection of flat feely bags that needed organising into some kind of toy. The best idea seemed to be to join them all together along one side and turn them into a strange kind of book.

At her next visit to the toy library, the little girl was given her special book—now enclosed in an eye-catching cover. We watched her explore it on her own. She scrunched up the pages, flicked them over, peered at the contents, waved the book about and generally showed her appreciation by playing with it for some considerable time. Satisfaction all round!

Self-help Rustly Book

Quick

A book for children must give pleasure, but it should also be informative and thought provoking. The Rustly Book seemed to satisfy the first requirement, but it might be interesting to try extending the idea. The next book could be more like a real one, telling a story or, at least, indicating a chain of events.

The purpose of the Self-help Rustly Book was to illustrate, in tactile and visual form, the routine of washing, brushing teeth and combing hair. The book had three pages made in bubbly plastic. A face flannel and a soap dish with a lid (containing strongly perfumed soap) were stitched to the first page. (Small holes were drilled in the base of the dish.) On the second were a toothbrush and an empty tube of toothpaste, still with its screw-top lid which could be removed for the child to smell the remains of the toothpaste. A comb was stitched to the third page and, alongside it, was a strip of ribbon stitched down at both ends. This held slides and bows which could be removed and used to adorn the child's hair.

A Book of Feely Trails

Long-lasting

This cardboard book was made for Tina, a little girl of six who had recently become blind. As her home tutor, it was up to me to show her how to use her fingertips for gathering information. Quite soon she would need this skill when she began to learn Braille. Inspiration eluded me, but then I remembered seeing at an International Conference of Toy Libraries some attractive mazes for children with severe visual impairment. These were mounted as a wall display but, in use, each one could be played with individually. Each maze was made of string, stitched to a backing of felt, which was then mounted on stiff cardboard to make a tile measuring about 20cm (8") square. The string meandered over the surface of the tile, never crossing over itself, but making an interesting pattern—perhaps forming a spiral, or a staircase, or a snake that curved from side to side. One of the features of each maze was that the beginning was indicated by a bead. Trace the string through to the end, and there was a button (like a full stop) to show you the finish. The mazes were attractive and had obviously been well used. Here was the inspiration I needed.

I began the book of feely trails for Tina. First, I needed the pages. Rectangles of sturdy card about A4 size seemed suitable. A visit to the local stationers produced some large split rings with hinges which would be ideal for holding the pages together. I planned to decorate the pages one by one, and gradually form them into a book, keeping the successful ones and learning from my mistakes!

The first page was quickly made from strips of fur fabric, arranged in lines, with the pile running from left to right. As with the mazes above, the starting point was indicated by a bead, and the finish by a button. This plan was followed throughout the book. Page two was a simple curly trail starting at the top left-hand corner and snaking its way down the page to the button at the bottom right-hand corner. It was formed by a line of finely crushed eggshells which would be slightly scratchy to follow and would, I hoped, encourage a light touch. The crushed eggshell was sprinkled on a line of adhesive, like glitter. Page three was the start of a series of string mazes, which became more complicated as Tina's skill increased. The split ring binding for the gradually expanding book was a useful way of keeping the pages together. They need not always be in the same order. I could introduce surprise pages and remove the boring ones when the book was too full.

The book of feely trails led on to various tactile books illustrating stories we shared, or 'Guess What?' pages, where Tina had to try to identify what I had stuck to the page—perhaps a hinged card teapot, which she could lift up and smell the teabag underneath. When inspiration failed, I fell back on some geometric shapes cut from sandpaper.

Tactile Story Books with a Magic Touch

Quick

Mary Digby,
Play Specialist,
Moorfields Eye Hospital

On our toy library shelves, you will find a few tactile books with pictures I have made from fabrics with interesting textures. These are fine as far as they go, but I have a feeling they sometimes appeal to the parents more than to the children! Mary Digby found a way to lift the whole idea of a tactile book onto a more child-centred plane. She and her students made books that related to *real life* situations. They were illustrated with *real* things that could be touched, and sometimes smelt, as the story unfolded. Each book contained several pages, and told about a little girl called Jenny, who did ordinary things like 'Visiting Granny'. In that particular story, page 1 described her being smartened up for the occasion. Alongside the writing, the page contained a *flannel* and *soap*, *Noddy toothbrush*, *nailbrush* and *comb*. All these were stuck, with Araldite, to the thick cardboard page. In spite of much handling, they are still there!

On page 2 Jenny's mother made her own preparations. She gave Jenny her spectacles to clean while she packed her handbag for the day. She put in her diary, watch, handkerchief, purse with money in it, and a bunch of keys. All these were mounted on the page.

By page 3 she had finished her preparations and taken the rollers out of her hair, put in her hair clips, chosen a necklace to wear and applied her perfume.

Page 4 described Jenny playing with a Bendy Doll while she waited for her mother. During her play, a button fell off her coat.

By page 5 they had arrived at Granny's. They walked over the pebbles on the path, smelled the lavender bush and examined the sea shells round the door before they rang the bell.

On page 6 Granny noticed the missing button. She found her thimble, needlebook and thread. She took her glasses out of their case and sewed on the button.

Now it was time for lunch, so Jenny laid the table with a knife, fork, spoon and paper plate. She arranged the plastic flowers to put in the middle.

The final page was all about going home. Granny, true to type, gave Jenny some goodbye presents: a balloon, some sweets and a pen.

In another volume, Jenny visited Moorfields Eye Hospital and she was introduced to the daily routine, the toys on the ward and the games the children liked to play. Further pages showed the toilet articles on the locker, and the equipment used before Jenny went to the operating theatre. Breakfast the next day would include an individual pack of Rice Krispies, a bendy straw and a sachet of tomato ketchup! After details of the morning's treatment, the book ended on a happy note with a picture Bingo board and all the cards to match to it and, of course, the Lucky Bag prize for winning!

Other titles included 'Jenny Goes to a Birthday Party', 'Jenny spends a night at Granny's House', and

'Jenny Goes on Holiday to Hungary'. This last one described in detail the flight and the experience of staying in an hotel.

With all the lumpy articles stuck to each page, these books were obviously very thick. The stout cardboard pages had holes punched in one side and were tied together with string.

SOME TOYS AND ACTIVITIES TO ENCOURAGE THE USE OF HANDS

A Simple Posting Box with Only One Hole

Instant

This toy can be a winner for any child who is just starting to take an interest in putting one thing inside another. This can happen at any age from about ten months upwards. As well as being good fun, cheap, and easy to make, this simple posting box makes a good introduction to more complicated commercial ones.

All you need is a tin with a plastic lid and a supply of cotton reels to post inside. The tin should be as large as possible. Make sure the lip is 'rolled' (not sharp) and that the cotton reels are all the same size. Use one as a template to mark a circle in the centre of the lid. Cut this out—with scissors, or with a heated needle embedded in a cork, so that you can hold it comfortably. The hole should be slightly larger than the reel, so that it will drop through easily. Check there are no jagged edges to the circle. (A rub with sandpaper will remove them.)

To make this simple toy more attractive, paint the tin and reels with Humbrol enamel. One coat should be sufficient, and you will end up with an attractive and colourful toy with twice the child appeal.

At the Sense Centre (for deaf/blind children) the teachers use a series of simple one hole posting boxes. They consider the special needs of the children with flaccid hands. The hole in the lid is made slightly smaller than the object to be posted, so that pushing it through the hole requires some effort. The children begin with a ping-pong ball. When they are successful, the ping-pong ball falls into the tin with a satisfying clonk. As they become adept at this, they

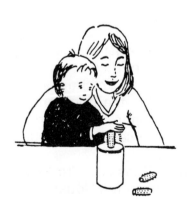

move on to another tin with a smaller hole which will just accept a wooden bead. Next comes a third for posting plastic hair curlers. These present a new problem. They need to be up-ended before they will fit into the hole. The sound and feel of the little plastic bristles on the sides of the curlers rubbing against the edge of the hole can set the teeth of an adult on edge but, of course, the children love it!

Posting Acorns in a Bottle

Instant

Susan Myatt,
Parent,
Kingston-upon-Thames
Toy Library

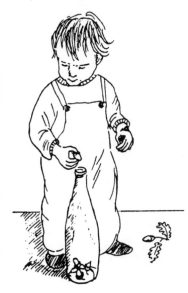

All children love to play with natural objects and things from the adult world. These are the nuts and bolts of our environment, and through them children learn about the world in which they live. Picture in your mind's eye a two-year-old totally absorbed in fitting the lids on heavy saucepans. A year later, he may be splashing in the puddles or scuffing up the Autumn leaves, while at home his big sister is playing at weddings, draping herself in an old net curtain and wearing her mother's shoes. Some children cannot share in these delights, but *if* you are reading this in the Autumn, and *if* you live near an oak tree, and *if* your child has reached the 'posting' stage, here is a chance to bring the outside world nearer to him, and let him practise his new-found skill into the bargain—and all completely free!

All you need is a bag full of acorns (perhaps you can collect them together) and a plastic bottle. If you want your child to practise fine finger movements, choose a bottle with a neck just wide enough to accept an acorn on end. Now sit back and watch his delight as he sees the bottle gradually filling up because of his own skilful efforts.

A Tropical Aquarium

Long-lasting

Mr Poediangga

As a student, Mr Poediangga attended a course at HEARU (Handicap, Education and Aids Research Unit) and invented this clever stacking toy.

Three chunky fish locate over short lengths of dowel fitted into a base board. (For even more stability, this can be clamped to the table.) The thickness of the wood makes the pieces easy to handle and, of course, each fish is attractively painted in brilliant tropical colours.

Materials
- A base board, say 350 × 150 × 20mm (14″ × 6″ × ¾″).
- Three short lengths of dowel, rounded at the top.
- Wood glue.
- A piece of 38mm (1½″) soft wood for the fish.
- Paint.
- Polyurethane varnish for protection.

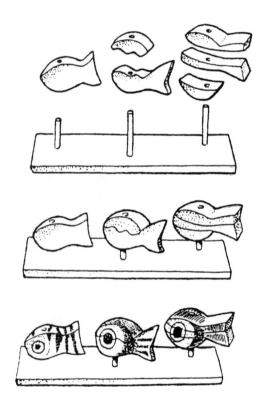

Method
Look at the illustration and drill holes in the base board for the dowel rods. Glue them in place. Cut out the outlines of the fish. Drill a hole through each, slightly larger than the diameter of the dowel for an easy fit. Leave one fish intact, divide the second into

two pieces and the last one into three. Sandpaper all the pieces. Paint them as gaudily as possible, then cover with at least two coats of polyurethane varnish.

The Peg Bus

Long-lasting

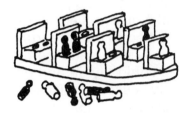

This was originally made in a workshop for adults with learning difficulties. It has been copied many times, and is a firm favourite with the children of three and upwards who come to our toy library. The bus is meant to represent a mini-bus, with the driver in front and the passengers sitting in pairs behind him. The seats have holes drilled in them. These are slightly wider than the pegs and fairly deep to allow the passengers to fit in easily and securely. The pegs are coloured in pairs, so that the toy can also be used for colour matching—the two yellow ones sharing the same seat. (The driver wears a white coat.) The bus is not fitted with wheels. This not only simplifies the construction, but prevents the bus from moving just as a peg man might be put in a hole.

Threading

Threading is a peaceful activity with many useful spin-offs. It encourages the use of both hands as well as hand-eye coordination. Other skills, such as colour matching, sorting or grading, can also become part of it. Leaving aside all these worthy attributes, most children at some stage in their lives really *enjoy* threading beads!

First of all, the skill of poking the threader through the hole must be learnt.

● In an Australian toy library the children begin by threading large haircurlers onto a length of plastic pipe.
● At Lekotek Korea, they use blocks of wood with holes bored through them and a piece of dowel to use as a threader. As the child's skill increases, bricks with smaller holes are provided.
● At some toy libraries in the UK, the children follow Roy McConkey's suggestion and thread plastic rings, cut from a washing-up liquid bottle, over a broom handle.

• Threading toys are, of course, available from toy shops. One is a set of plastic leaves with holes in them. By using the threaders provided, the veins on the leaves can be outlined. There are more ideas in the educational catalogues listed on p. 4 or here is a threading toy you can make yourself.

The Bee in a Tree

Long-lasting

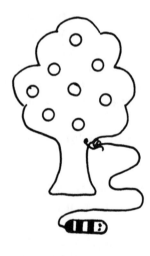

This delightful threading toy first appeared in the 'Making Toys' programme televised by the BBC in 1975. Its designer, David Chisnell, created a plywood tree shape, which had several holes drilled in the leafy part. A length of cord was tied to the tree trunk and, on the other end, was a busy bee made from a short length of dowel. The bee could 'fly' in and out of the holes until all the string was used up. This toy had a practical feature. The bee was attached to it, so could not be dropped or lost!

Materials
• *Either* an old table tennis bat with the rubber face removed, *or* a small piece of good quality ply, 5mm or 7mm, for the tree.
• About 5cm (2") of dowel for the bee, (longer rather than shorter) or you could use a long, fat macrame bead.
• A length of thin cord, say 20–30cm (8–12") or longer, depending on how far the child in question can stretch. Blind cord is best. This will not kink.
• An electric jig-saw or fretsaw.
• A large drill for making holes for the bee to fly through, and a very small one for the hole in the back of the bee and for attaching the cord to the tree.
• A dab of strong adhesive and a matchstick (for fixing the cord in the hole in the bee).
• Sandpaper.
• Paint, and polyurethane varnish for protection.

Method
Draw a tree shape on the plywood as suggested in the illustration. Shape out the bottom of the tree trunk to make it easier to grasp. Cut out the tree. Drill

holes at intervals in the leafy part. Drill a small hole in the trunk for the cord. Clean up all the rough edges with sandpaper. Round off the ends of the dowel (with sandpaper) and drill a small hole in one end to take the cord. Paint both sides of the tree green, with a brown trunk. Paint the bee yellow with black stripes. Protect all the paint with two coats of polyurethane varnish. Tie one end of the cord to the tree. Squirt some glue into the hole in the bee and poke in the other end of the cord. A needle is helpful to feed it in. Wedge it firmly in place with a small piece of matchstick coated with glue.

Making a Necklace

It takes a steady hand to hold a bead in position and aim a threader through the hole in the middle. Avoid the frustration (and possible bad temper) that can happen if beads roll out of reach, or the threader will not go through the hole easily. Here are some tips to consider.

1. Provide a container for the beads. A plastic cereal bowl is ideal. If keeping it upright or in one place is a problem, fix it to the table with a blob of Blu-tac, or a loop of masking tape.

2. Make sure the threader will go right through the bead and out the other side. Sometimes a round shoelace will do the job, but large beads may need a special threader available from educational suppliers. Nearer to hand is the polypropylene clothes line—the thin one without a wire core, used for whirly lines. This goes through the large holes in wooden beads very successfully, and is stiff enough to come well out of the hole for easy grasping and pulling through. Jewellers sell nylon threaders with a stiff wire end, which are excellent for older children who wish to thread small beads.

3. Brightly-coloured wooden beads can be bought at most toy shops. Square ones will not roll away and are easier to hold than round ones, which can easily slip through the fingers. Attractive adult beads which appeal to older children can often be bought at charity shops, car boot sales, etc.

DRESSING SKILLS

Buttons, Poppers and Zips

Children who are new to poking buttons through buttonholes will need the buttons to stand away from the cloth on a little stalk. To make the stalk, cross two pins (or place a matchstick) over the top of the button and sew over them as you attach the button to the cloth. Remove the pins and, to make the stalk, wind the thread round a few times between the bottom of the button and the cloth. Fasten off securely.

Scenes and Faces

Long-lasting

Monica Taylor,
Toy Librarian,
The Rix Toy Library

Monica makes colourful and motivating pictures where buttons play an essential part in the design. They may be needed to attach separate items to a picture or they might be used to complete a face. The pictures can be played with on the floor or table. With all the pieces in place, the larger ones hang on the wall as an attractive decoration. She has found them particularly useful for a little group of children with Down's Syndrome, but they are so colourful and attractive that everyone wants to have a go.

Supposing Monica wants to make a country scene. She will start with a background of calico and stitch to this a tree, a hill and some grass, cut from felt or any suitable material. Next, she attaches buttons (perhaps of different sizes) in strategic places, ready to receive the colourful felt shapes—each with a button hole—which will bring the picture to life. These are all made in felt, reinforced and stiffened with iron-on Vilene, and could be in the shape of birds, butterflies or apples to attach to the tree, or perhaps some rabbits and flowers for the grassy hill.

The faces, human or animal, are made slightly differently. Monica cuts two layers of fabric, face-shaped, and stitches them together at the top. On the top layer she makes button holes in the right position for the eyes, nose and mouth and adds hair, ears, whiskers, etc. as appropriate. On the bottom layer she stitches suitable buttons to be threaded through the holes and so complete the face.

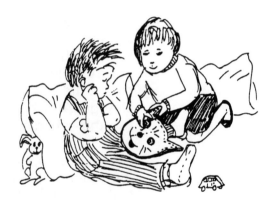

Inspired by Monica, I have also tried my hand at button pictures. These began as a series of button trainers I made for children with learning difficulties. At first they were like a simple rag book with only two pages, similar to Monica's button faces, turned on their sides. The buttons were stitched to the second page, and were threaded through the first. This idea was quite successful. There were no loose parts to be lost but, as I increased the number of buttons on the second page, it became obvious that the ones near the spine were quite difficult to manipulate. To overcome the problem, I made the next button trainer circular in shape. Using a dinner plate as a template, I cut two circles of fabric, and joined them together with a small circle of stitches in the centre. The most attractive buttons I could find were stitched to the unattached part of the bottom circle, and could be easily threaded through the holes in the top one.

This button circle was all very well in its way, but like my button books, I felt it was *boring*! It reminded me of a plate shape—after all that was its origin!—so I thought of a way of adding some food. I used some odd scraps of ply to cut out 'buttons' representing a full English breakfast! Now a fried egg, sausages, mushrooms, tomatoes, and bacon could all be threaded through their respective holes to fill the plate!

Car Button Trainer

Long-lasting

On the same principle of two pages, buttons on the second, a picture on the first, I have made a button trainer which has found favour with many of the toy library children. On the first page is a stitched picture of a child sitting in a car, waiting for the lights to change. Attached to the second page are the buttons for the wheels, the steering wheel, the car door (which opens) and the traffic lights. This simple scene seems to motivate even the most reluctant 'buttoners'! Every time the picture is given to a child—with the buttons not threaded through—their fingers get busy. In no time the car is compete with its wheels in place, and all the other buttons soon follow suit. It has well repaid the two evenings it took to make.

Button Snake

Long-lasting

This peculiar reptile is just a series of cloth segments, reducing in size from head to tail, each buttoning to the one in front. As the buttons are arranged in pairs, the segments are easy to link up in the right order.

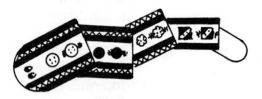

Materials
- Buttons—number of pairs and size according to the ability of the children.
- Fabric, for top pieces and linings.
- Button thread.
- Card or paper for a pattern.

Method

Draw patterns for the segments, the largest (i.e. for the head and following segment) about 10 × 14cm (4 × 5½"). Make the pattern for the next segment about 1½ cm narrower and shorter, and so on all down the line. Put the patterns on the wrong side of the fabric and draw round them. Cut *outside* the pencil lines. (They come in handy later as a stitching guide.) Round off the head and tail. Lay all the components out in front of you—top pieces, linings and pairs of buttons. You will see from the illustration that the head and tail have only one button each. All the other segments have two—the first to button to the segment ahead and the second (a dummy) to match the one that follows. Sew all the buttons to the top pieces. Then, beginning with the head, sew the top piece to its lining by putting right sides together, stitching most of the way round. Turn it right side out and close the opening. (Top stitch or oversew.) Make the button hole. Repeat the process all the way down the snake, remembering to adjust the size of the button hole as appropriate.

Popper Dollies

Long-lasting

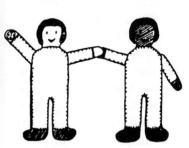

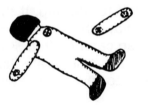

These little people are designed to give a child plenty of practice in pressing together the two parts of a press stud, or 'popper'. They are made from two layers of felt, stiffened with heavy duty iron-on Vilene. Their arms are attached to their bodies with press studs, and there is half another stud sewn to the back of one hand, with the opposite half stitched to the front of the other. With this arrangement, the little people can hold hands and be linked together in a friendly circle (or row).

The colours chosen represent the colours of the rainbow, (red, orange, yellow, green, blue, purple,) plus black and white. The dolls can have their arms arranged in different positions, or even interchanged, so that the yellow doll has red sleeves. If you have the stomach for it, remove all the arms, and jumble them up. Now the children can match up the colours and return them to their rightful owners, getting plenty of practice in 'popping' on the way.

LOOK AT IT THIS WAY

Australian Cushion

Quick

Take a tip from the Handbook of the Australian Association of Toy Libraries and make a special cushion covered with all sorts of fastenings. Remove the zip from an old pair of trousers; buttons and button holes from the front of a discarded dress; lacing holes from a worn-out canvas shoe; find an old belt with a buckle and sew them all firmly to a washable cushion cover. Put the cushion inside, rest it on the table or the child's knee and all the fastenings will be easy to reach. Children react favourably to this trainer, because it contains a variety of fastenings from *real* clothes. Maybe they will recognise the fancy buttons from the front of Auntie Mary's blouse!

Surprise Pockets

Quick

This is an easily made trainer which can be useful with a group of children who need to practise their fastenings. If several are made, each child can have a strip of pockets to explore, and next session she can try another one. In shape, this trainer is similar to a long envelope which has been divided into several sections, or pockets. The flap of the envelope makes the covering for the tops of the pockets and stops the (motivating!) surprises hidden inside from falling out. To lift the flap and find the surprise, a child must first tackle the fastening—Velcro, zip, button or popper.

The easiest way to make the pockets is to start off with a rectangle of material say 20 × 26cm (8 × 10½"). Make a hem all round the edge. Put the material wrong side up on the table. Turn the bottom edge up about 10cm (4") and machine over the hems at the sides to make the long envelope shape with a flap. Lift up the flap, and divide the bag part of the envelope into three pockets by running two rows of stitches from the folded bottom edge to the hem at the top. Sew half a fastening to the front of each pocket and the corresponding half to the flap. If the pockets are made this simple way, the fastenings must *all* be undone before the flap can be lifted. It is a more time-consuming job to attach a separate flap to each pocket, but if you are used to sewing that will be no problem for you.

I used a set of these pockets to good effect with a small group of slow learners. I had a box full of toys for the surprises—a tiny doll in a matchbox, a little plastic car, a homemade scrapbook, a few marbles, a toy watch to wind up and a doodle bag with a squeaker inside. I tried to add to the surprises each week. The children understood that the toys were not for keeping, but that they were entitled to play with them there and then, and the quicker they mastered the fastenings, the longer they would have to play! Each child chose a strip of ready-filled pockets, and was eager to discover what was inside. Before the session ended, they all returned their toys to the box and chose another set to replace them. These were put in the pockets and the fastenings happily *done up* again ready for the next session.

A Bag Full of Surprises

Long-lasting

Mrs Mackee,
Physiotherapist working
with visually impaired
children

In the course of her work, Mrs Mackee pays many home visits. As part of her stock in trade, she has made herself a large tote bag in brightly-coloured sail cloth. The bag is circular and has a firm base. (Thick cardboard, covered with material. It can be removed when the bag needs washing.) Both inside and out, the bag has many patch pockets of different sizes in which various toys can be hidden. For young children, these pockets can be made of different textures so that they are easy to identify. (For the tiny teddy bear look inside the fur fabric pocket!) Older children have to solve a problem before they can find a surprise. Some of the pockets close with Velcro—easy to prise apart—others need buttons, zips (with pull tags each end) or poppers to be undone before they will reveal their hidden treasures.

The children love this bag. The fun is not only in opening all the little pockets. At the end of playtime they seem to find it equally diverting to replace all the toys and secure them in their pockets for the next child to discover.

111

Life-sized Baby Dolls

Long-lasting

Fran Whittle and her team,
All Saints Arts and
Youth Centre, Sussex

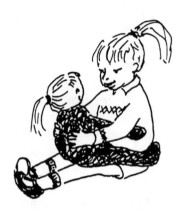

Toys and trainers that help children to manipulate fastenings definitely have their uses, but they are no substitute for the real thing. Fran's dolls can be dressed in proper clothes complete with zips, buttons, poppers and bows, and so help children to practise fastenings in a more lifelike situation.

Materials

- A Babygro, outgrown perhaps, or from the local jumble or car boot sale.
- Stretch fabric for the head, Fran recommends cotton stockinette.
- Polyester stuffing—with the CE safety mark on the pack.
- Wool, felt and thread for hair and features.

Method

First stuff the Babygro. Next make the head. Cut a strip of stretch fabric approximate for the size of the Babygro. (A young baby's body is about 3½ times the length of its head, and its neck is very short.) Stitch the short sides of the stretch fabric together to make a ring of material. Run a thread along one edge, gather up and fasten off securely. This is the top of the head. Turn the material inside out. Run another thread around the open (neck) end, unthread the needle and leave the thread dangling. Stuff the head, re-thread the needle, draw up the running thread and again fasten off securely. Put the head on top of the Babygro and join them together with several rounds of stitching. The doll will have a floppy head, just like a real baby. This makes it very appealing.

To make the face, first cut the features out of felt. Start with the eyes. These should be half way down the head (or slightly lower) and fairly wide apart. Pin them roughly in place. Do the same with the mouth (and nose?). Then try moving the pieces about a little to see how the expression changes. When you are satisfied, stitch the pieces in place and remove the pins. The hair can be made of wool. One method is to wind it over a piece of stiff paper and machine it down the middle. Cut the wool where it bends round the edges of the paper and tear the paper away.

Consider the row of stitching to be the parting and stitch firmly to the head along this line. Trim off any straggle ends. Select some suitable clothes (with lots of fastenings on them!) from the 'cast offs', and your doll is ready for tender loving care!

Sock Dollies

Quick

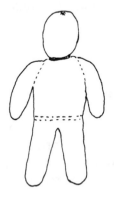

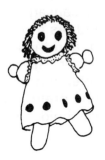

These cuddly little dolls are wonderful as 'extras' for imaginative play. If your child is short of patients for the shoebox hospital beds, here is a quick—and cheap—way to make good the deficit. If you take time to make the clothes removable, you provide yet another opportunity to provide practice in coping with fastenings.

Cut the foot off a sock and reserve this to make the arms. Think of the rest of the sock as being in three sections—head, body and legs. Pin where you think the neck and hips will be. First make the legs. Lie the sock flat on the table and cut through two thicknesses of material, from the ankle end to just below the pins that mark the hips. Round off the tips of the feet. Take out the pins. Turn the sock inside out and stitch up the bottoms of the feet and the inside leg seams. Do this very securely—two rows of stitching—and oversew the raw edge, otherwise the sock may fray easily and your seams could pull away. Turn the sock right side out. Stuff the legs with polyester fibre, and stitch across the body just above the top of the legs. This helps the dolly to sit down. Stuff the body section and tie (or gather) round the neck. You now have half a doll, with legs and a plump little body, but as yet no head or arms. Run a thread round the top of the sock. Stuff the head and draw up the thread. Fasten off very firmly. Cut two arms from the reserved sock foot. Round off the hand ends and sew them into sausage arms. (Strong seams as before.) Stitch the arms to the body very firmly. Sew on felt features, (or embroider them,) and add wool hair. Cover the head with large French knots for a curly hair style. For a straight cut, wind wool over some thin card, machine or hand stitch down the middle to keep the strands of wool in order. Cut the wool where it bends over the card. Tear the card away from the stitching. Sew the wool

113

hair to the doll, arranging the stitching along the line of the parting.

Make some simple dolls' clothes and play can begin.

The undressed sitting-down doll illustrated was made by a nine-year-old. She used the heel of the sock for the doll's sit-upon and cut the legs from part of the foot. She used the rest of the foot to make the arms, and folded down the top of the leg to make the cosy hat.

TACTILE GAMES

Tactile Ring Game

Long-lasting

This game was invented as a 'trainer' for the party game of 'Pass the Parcel'. A series of large fabric sausages, each with a different filling inside, were joined together with a length of piping cord between each, to form a ring. The children sat in a circle round the ring, and fiddled with the sausage in front of them. Then the music started, the sausages were passed from child to child until the music stopped. Pause for another fiddle with a different sausage until the music began again, and the sausages were once more passed from hand to hand. As a co-operation game for very young children, and those with learning difficulties, this one is a winner. The ring of sausages makes a good focus of attention and the different 'feels' (or noisemakers if you prefer) inside each as they rotate round the circle hold the children's interest.

Materials
- Different fabrics for the sausages. Strong, brightly coloured, perhaps textured, but not too thick or the contents cannot be felt. Size approx. 30cm (12") square.
- Lengths of piping cord for linking the sausages together. Approx. 36cm (14") long.
- Contents for the sausages, *see* lists on pp. 68 or 89 for inspiration.

Method

Decide on the number of sausages that you need, possibly six to eight. The number of children in the group you have in mind will be the deciding factor. You need one sausage per child and perhaps a couple of spare ones. Cut out the required number of squares of fabric and corresponding lengths of piping cord. Turn in the ends of each sausage and hold down with gathering thread. Stitch the sides of the sausage together. (Two rows of stitching advised, for strength.) Tie a *large* knot at each end of a length of piping cord. Put one knot inside the sausage. Gather up the end and use the thread to stitch the cord (just above the knot) firmly in place. Insert contents into the sausage. Gather up as before and stitch firmly. You now have a tactile sausage with piping cord protruding from each end. Repeat the process with another sausage, and add it to a cord from the first one. Continue in this way until the ring is complete. Now all you need is a circle of children to appreciate your efforts!

Tabletop games

Mary was a little girl who had recently lost her sight. As her home tutor, it was up to me to help her through the difficult period of adjustment. I needed to make, and sometimes invent, a variety of tactile games which would help her to 'think' through her fingertips. When the time came for her to learn Braille, sensitive fingertips would be essential. We began with adaptations of traditional dominoes and lotto games described in the chapter on 'Learning to Look'.

Tactile Dominoes

Quick

In this game, textures (from the list on p. 91) replaced the normal dots. Tactile dominoes are available commercially, but the tactile areas—presumably for reasons of cost—are always on the small side. This is fine for children who are already used to gaining information through their fingertips, but younger children and those, like Mary, who have been in the habit of using their eyes rather than their fingers, need a larger area to feel. Make your own set of dominoes and the sky is the limit!

Mary's set of tactile dominoes were made from eight rectangles of thick card, each 10 × 20cm (4 × 8"). I drew a line down the centre of each and arranged the rectangles in a line. Then the fun began! The left-hand half of the first rectangle was left blank. Adhesive was smeared, right up to the edges, on the right-hand half, and on the left-hand half of the second rectangle. Both these sticky sections were covered with velvet. The process was repeated with the right and left halves of the second and third rectangles—this time using sandpaper—and so on all along the line, finishing with a blank.

In play, we would each have four rectangles. In turn, one of us would start the game by putting a rectangle on the table. The other player would hope to find a matching texture among her collection. If no luck, a turn was missed. Ultimately, all the textures would be needed. The sequence of textures was always the same, but it could begin and end in a different place, which added a little variety to the game.

Button Dominoes

Long-lasting

Here buttons of distinctive shapes were substituted for textures. They were sewn to rectangles of double felt, and made a more difficult game than the one above.

Materials
- Felt.
- Iron-on Vilene for stiffening.
- Button thread for attaching the buttons firmly.
- As many different pairs of buttons as is suitable for the child in question. For young children use large buttons with very distinctive shapes, and not too many pairs. At a later stage the game can, of course, be made more challenging by introducing more pairs and smaller buttons.

Method
Back the felt with iron-on Vilene. Cut out twice the number of rectangles, say 10 × 5cm (4 × 2"), required

for your game. Half will hold the buttons, the rest will back them, adding extra stiffness, and covering the stitches which attach the buttons. Arrange the buttons in the usual domino sequence—right-hand side on one rectangle corresponding to the left-hand side of the next. Stitch the buttons on firmly. Add the backing pieces, stick and stitch.

Note
These dominoes will hand wash, but don't put them in with the clothes in case the colour runs.

Another set of these button dominoes was made for three children with severe visual impairment, but we had a problem. As they played together, it was almost impossible for them to keep the dominoes in line. The solution was easy, thanks to our good friend Velcro! A strip, long enough to hold the line of dominoes was stuck and stitched to felt. This was mounted on a strip of stiff cardboard to give it stability. The other half of the Velcro was cut to size, and sewn to the backing pieces before they were stuck and stitched to the button layer.

Real Things Dominoes

Long-lasting

A school for severely visually impaired children near to me needed new toys to add to their toy library.

I remembered seeing a set of Real Things Dominoes designed by Roger Limbrick. The items on his dominoes included hinges, buttons, keys, nylon scouring pads, corks, doorknobs, pencils, metal letters, sliding bolts, bell push buttons, keyhole plates, detergent bottle tops, etc. This list is sufficient to give you the idea.

Materials
- Plywood or medium density fibreboard, say 12mm.
- Pairs of objects to attach as suggested by the list above, and added to by you. I also included fluffy woolly balls, cotton reels and little toy cars—with their wheels removed so that they would lie flat.
- Very strong adhesive such as Araldite.

- Small screws to use as appropriate.
- Polyurethane varnish to protect the wooden parts.

Method

From the plywood or MDF cut out and sandpaper the required number of rectangles, say 15 × 7cm (6 × 3″). Lay out the dominoes in a row and arrange the 'real things' in the best order. Glue (and screw?) them in place. Cover the exposed parts of the wood with polyurethane varnish. As an extra refinement, a strip of Velcro can be stuck to both ends of the dominoes so that, in play, they can be coupled together and not joggled out of line.

Feely Bingo

Quick

This game is similar to ordinary Bingo, or Lotto, but (yes, you've guessed it!) textures replace the number or pictures. To make a game for three, you will need six fairly large sheets of stiff card, three for the master cards and three to cut up. Raid your rag bag for scraps of suitable material and consult the list on p. 91. Take a master card and stick on about four squares of contrasting textures—say sandpaper, fur fabric, velvet and lino tile. Repeat these textures on another card, and cut this one into four pieces, so that each can be matched to the ones on the master card. Repeat the process with the other cards, using different textures on each pair.

To play, all the small cards are placed face downwards in the middle of the table. Each player has a master card and takes it in turns to pick a small one from the centre. If it matches a texture on his card, he keeps it and puts it on the appropriate place. If it does not match, he returns it to the centre—and so on until all the cards are full.

Note

If a small card is lost the game is useless, so it is worthwhile, at the making stage, to provide a box or bag for all the pieces.

Using the sense of smell

THE SENSE OF SMELL IS PERHAPS THE LEAST *obviously* stimulating and useful of all the five senses, but it can give much pleasure and, for children with a visual impairment, it can also be extremely useful as a mobility aid. Imagine you know these two children. Michael is seven and has multiple disabilities. If a few drops of perfume are sprinkled on his pillow, he will make a big effort to turn his head to enjoy the smell. Mark is ten and attends a school for the visually impaired. During the holidays he often shops with his mother. He has never been known to confuse the butcher's shop with the baker's for he can confidently distinguish them by smell. He has learnt to trust his nose to confirm much of the information he receives through his ears and fingers. Between these two children with their special problems, there lies a huge group of others, each with their own personal difficulties. For all of them their lives can be enriched if they make the most of every sense—and that includes the sense of smell.

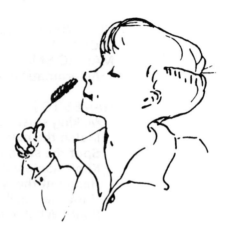

We notice when a baby has learnt to focus, because we see her stare at something interesting, or look into our eyes and smile back at us. We know she is aware of sounds when she turns her head to investigate a sound behind her. Her delight in her sense of touch is obvious when she starts to grasp, poke and stroke all the interesting textures she finds and, of course, at mealtimes she makes it crystal clear that some tastes please her more than others. The development of her sense of smell is less obvious. If you offer her a flower and invite her to enjoy its perfume she will probably wrinkle up her nose, but instead of sniffing will snort or snuffle! Perhaps she just lacks control over her breathing. By

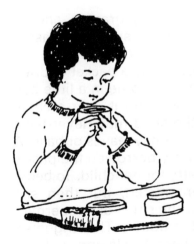

the time she has become fully mobile and increasingly skilful with her hands, she may discover that ecstatic experience of unscrewing the lids from her mother's cosmetic jars and we find her sniffing appreciatively at their pleasant perfumes. As she grows older, smells will have certain associations, will help to enrich her memories and perhaps even warn her of danger. Every adult has a mental catalogue of smells which has been built up over the years, and many of these will have been first experienced in childhood. Perhaps the smell of new leather shoes is associated with stiff, shiny sandals on the first day of the summer term, or the smell of mud flats at low tide with a happy holiday. When we think about smells, we realise we all have our own particular likes and dislikes, just as we do with sights, sounds, feels and tastes. Unless we provide our children with plenty of opportunities to explore and experiment, they will find it difficult to discover what they really like.

HELPING CHILDREN ENJOY THE SENSE OF SMELL

How can children with special needs be helped to develop and enjoy the sense of smell? Parents who hope to solve the problem by visiting a toy shop will find there are scarcely any smelly toys available. Smells are such transitory things, literally carried away on the wind, that any toy manufacturer, no matter how enterprising, would be hard put to it to add a universally acceptable and long-lasting one to his product. This means that those of us concerned with the play needs of the children who need our help must make a conscious effort to introduce some smells into their play—in the same way as we think about providing colour, sound and texture.

We can make use of activities and games which include different perfumes—some well-tried ones are described in this chapter—but perhaps the richest source of stimulating smells is the child's own environment. One imaginative teacher takes her non-ambulant children to lie in the long grass at the end of the school garden. Imagine the delight of

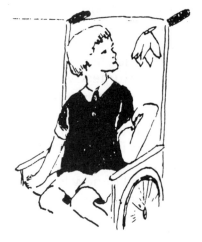

being surrounded by tall waving grasses and to smell the warm earth and the hay—surely a pleasant change from disinfectant and soap suds! In the winter the same teacher would buy a packet of dried herbs from the supermarket, put some in a little bag made from thin material, and hang it near a child. Without this forethought, the child may never have had the chance to smell mint or bay leaves or basil. A parent who uses our toy library borrowed the pastry kit and made some play pastry for her child. To begin with he was not at all interested, but then she remembered his passion for the smell of peppermint and added a few drops to the dough. That triggered his interest and he began happily playing with his special pastry, squeezing, prodding and rolling it, and finally chopping it into little pieces with a plastic paper knife.

It takes imagination and an empathy with the child to think of such ways of stimulating the sense of smell. Even the everyday experience of going shopping can be made into an exciting outing of aromatic discovery! Imagine you can watch the mothers in the two following situations and draw your own conclusions!

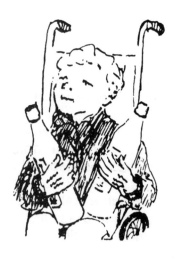

Mrs A. is going shopping with Peter who is four years old and has very little sight. She is in a hurry today, because her friend is coming to tea, and she has had a frustrating morning. The shops are not far away, but to save time she pops Peter in the buggy and walks there as quickly as possible, hurrying over her selection of food at the supermarket and remembering to buy the bottle of white spirit for her husband. On the way home her plastic bag is in danger of splitting with the weight of all her purchases, so she gives the white spirit and a bottle of lemonade to Peter to hold, one in each arm, as he sits in the buggy. When she reaches home, she takes them from him and Peter hears her put them on the kitchen table with the other shopping. She turns her attention to helping Peter with his coat and gloves, answers the 'phone and puts the buggy away. The door bell rings. It is the milkman calling for his money. Meanwhile, Peter fancies a drink of lemonade. He knows the bottle is on the table. He remembers it is tall and heavy because he nursed it all the way home. Confidently, he reaches on the shelf for his mug and places it on the draining board. He takes the nearest bottle, unscrews the lid and begins to pour. Luckily Mrs A. returns to the kitchen at that moment so disaster is averted!

Mrs B. is also going shopping, taking with her the baby and four-year-old Lucy who is without sight. Her shopping list is not long today; just white spirit, lemonade, toilet soap, fish and some parsley for the sauce. Lucy walks briskly along, holding on to the handle of the pram. She knows when she is nearly at the end of her road, because the man who lives in the last house has planted an evergreen hedge. This has a special smell and tickles her fingers as she drags them through the young bushes. The man is busy gardening. She can hear his shears cutting the grass border on the other side of the hedge. He calls a greeting and the shopping expedition is diverted through the front gate. He wants to show Lucy how well his herb garden is growing, so they all troop round to the side of the house. Here Lucy, (who can already identify sage, parsley and mint) is delighted to examine a little bush of rosemary, crushing a few leaves between her fingers to increase the smell. They go on their way, Mrs B. with a bag of parsley for the sauce, and Lucy with a little posy of herbs to plant in a saucer garden when she reaches home.

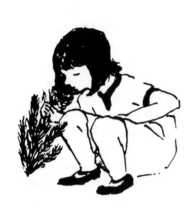

Further down the street, they pause to make way for the delivery man who is carrying a large tray of freshly-baked rolls into the baker's shop. They smell so good that Mrs B. and Lucy decide to buy some. Later, in the supermarket, Lucy helps to push the trolley to the corner where the coffee grinder is kept. Mrs B. selects the beans she wants, takes one out and gives it to Lucy to play with while the others are being ground. Before she seals down the bag, she gives Lucy the opportunity to feel the soft powder and to smell its particular fragrance. Now to buy the toilet soap. There is plenty of chance to sniff and compare here, and Lucy is allowed to choose the one she likes best. Mrs B. gropes in the freezer for the

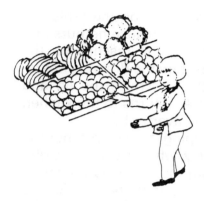

fish, and then adds the bottle of lemonade to the contents of the trolley. They make for the checkout nearest the greengrocery shelves. Many of the trays for the fruit and vegetables are at the edge of the shelf, just level with Lucy's nose. Without touching them, she can feel her way along the edge of the shelf and try to identify them by smell. Here are the apples, oranges and bananas. Next come cauliflowers, onions and earthy potatoes. Each time they play this game, Lucy becomes more sure of the answers.

They leave the supermarket and go to the iron-mongers. They find the manager arranging a new delivery of candles. He accidentally drops one. Quickly Lucy feels for it and holds it up for him. She is enjoying the sensation of wax against her hot little fingers which are rapidly exploring this fascinating object with its little tail of string. The lady who buys that candle may well wonder why it has tiny grooves all up one side!

Mrs B. buys the white spirit. The manager turns to help another customer and, while they wait to pay, Mrs B. realises she has just bought something poten-tially very dangerous, which is quite new to Lucy's experience. She tells her about the white spirit and that daddy will need it to clean his paint brushes. She lets her examine the bottle, then carefully removes the stopper so that she can sniff the dangerous liquid. She replaces the stopper, pays her bill and makes a great fuss of placing the bottle at the foot of the pram, well out of reach of the baby. The shop-ping now done, Mrs B. turns the pram towards home and a nice cup of coffee, fresh bread rolls and a refreshing drink of lemonade for Lucy.

MAKING SMELLS

Essences and perfumes can be made more manage-able by sprinkling them on a small pad of cotton wool or absorbent paper. Only use a very small amount of any essence, partly to avoid waste, but mainly because strong smells—even nice ones—can sometimes give a very unpleasant sensation; for example, eucalyptus oil, if smelt too vigorously, could discourage a child from ever sniffing again! Aim at an aroma rather than a smell. An easy way of producing this is to take only one or two drops from the bottle by poking in a drinking straw just below the surface of the liquid, then hold your finger firmly over the open end. Lift the straw from the bottle, hold it over the pad you want to perfume and take your finger away. The liquid will instantly fall where you direct it. Smells can be diluted by adding them to a damp pad. To make the pad easier to handle, put it in a tin with holes in the lid or wrap it in a square of cloth and tie it in.

Smells can be sprinkled on favourite soft toys or added to fabric collage such as the Feely Trail Along the Wall (p. 91). Next time you go to a jumble or car boot sale, look out for an old-fashioned scent spray. Put in a few drops of perfume and you have a new toy! Children love to use it to squirt smelly jets of air onto their faces—good practice in squeezing too! A substitute scent spray can be made very quickly from an empty plastic detergent bottle. Take off the nozzle, wash it and thoroughly rinse out the bottle to remove all traces of the detergent smell. Cut off and throw away the stopper and the little strip of plastic that joins it to the nozzle. Put a little cotton wool or a small piece of rag impregnated with your child's favourite perfume into the bottle and replace the nozzle. The puffer makes a very satisfactory toy for most children. For the inquisitive ones, you can fix the nozzle in place with a dab of polystyrene cement —sold for making up plastic model kits. This makes the toy perfectly safe for supervised use, but will not deter a child who is really determined to remove it.

An Aromatic Herbaceous Border

Quick

Margaret Gillman and Staff, White Lodge Centre

In this nursery unit for children with Cerebral Palsy the staff add colour and perfume to the classroom. They make tissue paper flowers with cotton wool centres, and sprinkle them with scent. When they are not being used for decorative purposes, a child may be given one to hold, or wear as an outsized button-hole. A child celebrating a birthday may have a garland of them draped round her wheelchair.

Each flower is made from a pipe-cleaner, a small ball of cotton wool and some tissue paper in eye-catching colours. Margaret gave me one as a sample, which I promptly vandalised to see how it was made! The dimensions given are for a flower *about* 14cm (5½") across. Make one to get the knack, then adjust the size as you wish.

Fold the pipe-cleaner in half. Push a cotton wool ball tightly against the bend and twist the pipe-cleaner to hold it firmly in the middle. Cut two different coloured squares of tissue paper about 14cm square. Lay one on top of the other and pleat them together, creasing them one way and then the other, zigzag fashion, as though you were making a fan. Keeping the pleats together, fold the paper in half. With scissors, round off the corners at the open ends. Still keeping the pleats together, open out the paper and push the central crease between the ends of the pipe-cleaner and hard against the cotton wool ball. Twist up the pipe-cleaner as tightly as possible to squeeze the tissue paper and hold it in place. Tease out the pleats until each half of the flower is like a semicircular fan. Join the edges of the fans together with a dab of glue. Bend up the sharp ends of the pipe-cleaner and bind them with masking tape. Lastly, sprinkle a few drops of perfume on the cotton wool.

GAMES TO PLAY WITH SMELLY BAGS

These games are suitable for individual children or small groups.

Making Smelly Bags

Instant

Make these from squares of old material. Wrap a cotton wool ball in each square and tie it up—like a bouquet garni! Liquids can be sprinkled on the cotton wool, or powders buried inside it. If possible, involve the children in the making of the smelly bags. This way they have the opportunity of handling the substance and associating it with its smell before it disappears inside the bag.

Match the Pairs

Instant

Make up two or three pairs of bags with the same smell and invite the child to pair them off.

Spot the Stranger

Quick

Collect a few film cartons and punch holes in the lids. Make the contents of them all smell the same—except for one. You might put lavender or pot pouri in the set and a squirt of toothpaste in the 'stranger'. The possibilities are endless!

Kim's Game with Smells

Quick

Place not more than five smelly bags (with identical covers) on a tray. The child sniffs and identifies each one. He hides his eyes and one bag is removed. He must then sniff all the bags again and try to name the missing one.

Hang Out the Washing

Quick

The child pegs smelly bags at wide intervals along a low-hung washing line—the bags about level with his nose. He must then 'bring in the washing' and fetch whichever smell he is asked for.

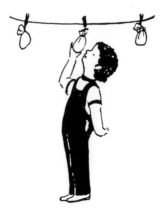

Hunt the Smell

Instant

This game is played like 'Hunt the Thimble', but a smelly bag is hidden for the child to find. (This is one occasion when you can be generous with the essence!)

All these games will only last for one session. If they are stored, all the smells will fade or combine—interesting perhaps, but useless as a scent discrimination game. One of the advantages of using film cartons is that they can be emptied and washed at the end of the session and refilled for the next time.

Pooh—What a Pong!

Some children love to concoct *bad* smells, perhaps combining peppermint essence with vinegar! All good fun, but make sure the ingredients in the concoction are safe—albeit obnoxious! It gives children the greatest pleasure to see an adult sniff such an evil concoction and pull a face over it!

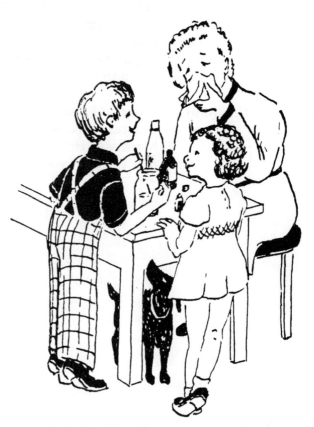

SMELLY GIFTS FOR CHILDREN TO MAKE

Lavender Bags

Children love making these, and they can be acceptable presents for relatives and friends. Any thin material is suitable for the bags, but one with small holes in it—like net curtaining—is nice, because the lavender can be seen inside.

The simplest lavender bag is made by putting a little pile of lavender in the centre of a square or circle of material. Gather the material round the lavender and tie up firmly with a length of ribbon. One little girl who spent many hours lying on her tummy liked to fill little bags like tiny pillow cases. She managed very well and had quite a production line going! She stripped the lavender from the stalk into a bowl. Then she shovelled it into a bag with a teaspoon, hardly spilling any. She tied up the bag with ribbon, then frayed out the top to make a decorative fringe.

Lavender Dolls

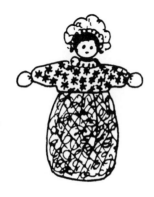

I like to make tiny brooch dolls with lavender bags as their skirts. These can be pinned to children who have severe disabilities. The child can enjoy the pleasant, delicate smell, and the brooch can serve as a talking point for any passing adult who is likely to remark upon it and stop for a chat with the child! I make a little head out of material from a pair of tights, stuffed with a scrap of polyester filling. This is inserted into a 'T'-shaped fabric torso. The skirt is made like the lavender bag above, and gathered to the torso. The features are embroidered and the head either covered with wool hair, or a little mob cap trimmed with lace. A safety pin is sewn to the back of the doll.

Pomanders

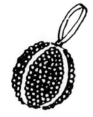

These make good Christmas presents, but need to be made in good time to allow them to dry out—so start early! Choose a well-shaped orange. Mark it vertically into four segments, with narrow strips of Sellotape. This shows where the ribbon will go and defines the sections to be filled with cloves. Using a fine knitting needle, or a cocktail stick, make a hole in the orange just deep enough to take a stalk of a clove. Push in a clove, then make another hole—and so on until every section is filled. (Do not squeeze the orange or the juice may dribble out.) Roll the pomander in ground cinnamon and wrap it in foil— or waxed paper from a cereal packet. Keep it in a warm cupboard for about six weeks while it dries out and shrinks. Finally, remove the Sellotape and tie the orange up with pretty ribbon.